Concentration and Choice in Health

Concentration and Choice in Healthcare

Edited by

Dr Brian Ferguson

Dr Trevor A. Sheldon

Dr John Posnett

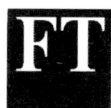

FT

FINANCIAL TIMES
Healthcare

FT HEALTHCARE
a Division of Pearson Professional Ltd
Maple House, 149 Tottenham Court Road, London
W1P 9LL, UK
Telephone: +44 (0)171 896 2424
Fax: +44 (0)171 896 2449
http://www.fthealthcare.com

First edition 1997

A catalogue record for this book is available from the
British Library

ISBN 0443 05939X

Publisher: John Harper
Project Manager: Brenda Wren
Copy edited by: Samantha Evans, Sawbridgeworth
Indexed by: Helen McKillop, Menstrie

Typeset by Saxon Graphics Ltd, Derby

Printed by Bell & Bain Ltd, Glasgow

Contents

Contributors

Vassilis Aletras
Aristotle University of Thessaloniki

Pauline Allen
London School of Hygiene and Tropical Medicine, and Brent & Harrow Health Authority

Richard J. Arnould
Department of Economics, Program in Health Economics, Management and Policy, University of Illinois

Roy Carr-Hill
Centre for Health Economics, University of York

Lawrence M. DeBrock
Department of Economics, Program in Health Economics, Management and Policy, University of Illinois

Robin Dowie
Health Economics Research Group, Brunel University

Jane Eminson
Chief Executive, Wolverhampton Health Authority

Brian Ferguson
Centre for Health Economics, University of York, and North Yorkshire Health Authority

Maria Goddard
Centre for Health Economics, University of York

Hugh Gravelle
National Primary Care Research and Development Centre, Centre for Health Economics, University of York

Andrew Jones
Department of Economics and Related Studies, University of York

Justin Keen
Department of Government, Brunel University

Peter Kennedy
Chief Executive, York Health Sciences Trust

Michael Place
York Health Economics Consortium, University of York

John Posnett
York Health Economics Consortium, University of York

Heather L. Radach
Department of Economics, Program in Health Economics, Management and Policy, University of Illinois

Trevor A. Sheldon
NHS Centre for Reviews and Dissemination, University of York

Amanda J. Sowden
NHS Centre for Reviews and Dissemination, University of York

Ian Watt
NHS Centre for Reviews and Dissemination, and Department of Health Studies, University of York

Acknowledgements

Much of the work required for this book has involved extensive literature-searching and the acquisition of documents from numerous and diverse sources. The editors would particularly like to thank Julie Glanville and Linsee Johnstone in the Centre for Health Economics (CHE)/NHS Centre for Reviews and Dissemination (CRD) Information Service at the University of York for their assistance in this respect. We would also like to thank the secretarial staff in CHE, CRD and the York Health Economics Consortium (YHEC) for their hard work in preparing material for publication.

A significant proportion of the book draws upon research which CHE, CRD and YHEC were commissioned in 1996 to undertake by the NHS Executive under the auspices of the 'Concentration and Choice' project. The idea for the book and subsequent contributions were stimulated by that project, and the editors acknowledge the considerable support and constructive criticism of Donald Franklin and Andrew Lloyd at the NHS Executive throughout the research. Finally, we would like to thank all the contributors who have made our task considerably easier through meeting various deadlines and through the quality of their contributions.

Brian Ferguson, Trevor A. Sheldon, John Posnett

1

Introduction

Brian Ferguson, Trevor A. Sheldon, John Posnett

Health services throughout the world are under pressure to concentrate the provision of hospital services and at the same time to decentralise and de-bureaucratise the organisation of healthcare. A primary-care orientation has been fostered in the UK NHS, with the aim of making healthcare more responsive to local needs within a 'patient-centred' approach. In the drive to promote efficiency and quality of care and to contain spiralling costs, most countries seem to be reforming their healthcare systems with both intended and unintended effects on the configuration of services. Price competition in countries with more market-orientated healthcare systems such as the USA has resulted in a system of hospital mergers, buy-outs and both horizontal and vertical integration. Similar results, the concentration of services in fewer and larger provider units, have also been achieved in more centrally controlled and regulated systems such as in the UK. There has also been a growth of 'big ticket' health technologies, which to be cost-effective need a larger catchment population than is served by smaller hospitals. These changes can have far-reaching effects on competition in the long run, with the danger of hospitals exploiting monopoly power and raising prices. There are also potentially adverse effects on access to services, especially for more vulnerable groups in society. These need to be set against the potential gains in efficiency and effectiveness achieved by concentrating and specialising services. Higher throughput, improvements in clinical expertise through carrying out more procedures, and exploitation of any economies of scale and scope may help keep costs in check whilst at the same time improving healthcare outcomes.

Unfortunately, healthcare reform often takes the form of a panic response to apparent crises, overly influenced by ideology and unchallenged assumptions about the wisdom of topical proposals. Such reform is frequently driven by the promise of system benefits given by international consultants or management gurus who peddle certainties. Given the profound effects of healthcare reforms in general and the concentration of hospital services in particular, it is important that healthcare policy-makers take a more systematic approach when considering regulatory and incentive structures which promote change. In particular, they should take into account and appraise critically the research evidence available on the factors which determine the efficiency and effectiveness of structures of healthcare delivery. This book explains some of the forces underlying changes in hospital provision, and considers the relevant international research evidence and its implications for decisions about the optimal scale and scope of hospitals.

Hospitals have often been viewed as factories, with healthcare professionals and health technologies being the inputs and either patient throughput or health gain being the output. Using this production-process model, the question arises whether the production process can be made more efficient by increasing scale. Can unit costs be reduced by spreading fixed costs over a greater number of patient episodes? Hospitals emerged partly because of the need to put together different skills when treating individual patients. The more disciplines which are needed to diagnose, treat and rehabilitate patients, the greater is the pressure to house them in one facility. Therefore, another question is whether by carrying out a broader range of activities in one hospital, more efficient use can be made of services or equipment that can serve a number of functions (economies of scope). A further question related to the production process concerns the possibility of increasing the quality of care (improved health gain and reduced risk of adverse outcomes) by increasing the size of a hospital in general, or more particularly by increasing the volume of any one set of procedures carried out by the hospital or clinician.

For example, do hospitals which carry out more coronary artery bypass graft operations, or clinicians who see more breast cancer patients, have better outcomes, and if so, is there an optimal level or minimum quality threshold? The more quality gains arising from increasing volume, the greater are the pressures to increase specialisation in healthcare. Specialisation (and super-specialisation) itself has its own in-built dynamic towards the centralisation and concentration of services and hence the size of units.

However, the industrial model of healthcare has limitations and the lessons from the industrial sector may not always be relevant. The 'production process' in healthcare is considerably more complex and patient care needs to be individualised to some extent. The uncertainty inherent in much clinical practice means that guidelines and protocols cannot be followed slavishly. We talk rarely of output but more often of outcomes, since the aim of healthcare is to improve a complex range of dimensions affecting people's quality of life and welfare. The benefits (and costs) may be experienced not just by individual patients but also by their families and the community at large. Since healthcare is viewed as a basic right and a 'merit good', society often has expectations of and places duties on hospitals which are of a higher order than those typically expected from service or manufacturing industries. We are, therefore, concerned to ensure that people in need have sufficient access to appropriate healthcare services. As a result health services are to differing extents funded publicly by some form of social insurance and are held accountable to the public. Changes in the structure of health services, the size of hospitals and the development of separate purchaser/ provider responsibilities all affect the concentration of power and control, with implications for the public accountability of health services. Justin Keen (Chapter 9) outlines the nature of arrangements for ensuring the accountability of the NHS to Parliament and discusses how changes in the healthcare system pose challenges for the mechanisms of accountability. If hospitals become highly concentrated, the market power of any one purchaser or commissioner is likely to be reduced and the notion of local accountability becomes somewhat unreal.

One element of public accountability is access, which may itself be affected by the concentration of hospitals into large and geographically more distant units. Any negative effects of concentration on utilisation, health and private costs (e.g. for travel) need to be set against any efficiency gains from larger units, taking into account the distribution of the impact on different social and client groups. In Chapter 4 Roy Carr-Hill and colleagues examine research evidence on the determinants of healthcare utilisation and the potential effects of service concentration on use. Overall it is found that utilisation of services does tend to decay with distance, and this may result in inappropriate delays in seeking care. This may shift some costs from the health sector onto individuals, which is likely to have more of a negative impact on those with less income and control over resources. The overall effects of this on levels of health are not clear and to a great extent may depend on the adequacy of primary care and referral decisions made by family physicians. Particular efforts might be best focused on countering the distance-decay in preventive programmes by encouraging early presentation and attendance for screening. One study has shown that positive systematic action such as a call-and-recall system improved use of a centralised screening programme in the UK. In addition, the costs of travel for low-income groups should be taken into account in appraisals of proposed service reconfigurations, in particular where the likely effect is to increase the distance of available services from some patients.

Healthcare markets even in the most *laissez-faire* economies are heavily regulated. In Chapter 9 Pauline Allen considers the legal framework of the NHS. Hospital Trusts, although operationally independent, are still publicly owned and much of their activity is controlled by central rules. The degree to which hospital concentration occurs in the NHS is still largely determined by a politically-influenced administrative hierarchy. The contradiction between this central control and the drive to promote competition and choice is discussed in detail by Maria Goddard and colleagues (Chapter 7) who consider the role of regulation in addressing some of the issues raised by concentration of services in the NHS. As in the case of utilities such as gas and electricity, there are elements which are (at least locally) likely to be naturally monopolistic and other activities which lend themselves to competition.

One of the roles of regulation is to ensure that potentially beneficial competition is promoted. In order to promote supply-side competition and contestability, the Department of Health produced guidance in 1994 on 'The Operation of the NHS Internal Market'. This provides a framework for the consideration of hospital mergers *inter alia* which takes into account likely market share and which makes reference to the issue of hospitals that 'fail'. However, the regulatory policy is rather discretionary and lacking in detail, thereby increasing uncertainty instead of providing a clear and explicit structure in which activity and transactions can occur. In this it mirrors the regulation of the privatised utilities in the UK, which can result in the regulators acting in the interests of the providers rather than the public. The discretionary nature of regulation in Britain can also result in political considerations over-riding those of efficiency. Thus, for example, it is possible that the local and national political costs of allowing public hospitals to close for financial reasons encourages hospital mergers as a more acceptable form of market 'exit', without a full examination of the underlying causes of the problem. The regulatory structure in the NHS will need to be changed whatever structural reforms are introduced by the new Labour Government. The power of those responsible for commissioning hospital services on behalf of the public could be strengthened as a counter-balance to increased provider concentration or as a means of influencing reconfigurations in supply. In Chapter 7 the authors consider where regulatory control should reside.

In the USA, the healthcare market is highly developed and so is the system of regulation. The last two decades have witnessed a rapid concentration of ownership and provision of services with high levels of vertical and horizontal integration. These developments are described and analysed by Richard Arnould and colleagues in Chapter 8. The introduction of greater, although highly regulated, competition in the early 1980s reduced costs and prices in competitive local hospitals because of the ability of Health Maintenance Organisations (HMOs) to steer patients to more efficient providers. Competition was facilitated by rigorous enforcement of the anti-trust laws (from which healthcare providers had been partly exempt) and a move to payer-driven healthcare. However, competition inevitably leads to concentration of provision especially in areas where market entry (setting up a new hospital) is difficult. In the USA, incentives have led to hospitals increasingly becoming owned by shareholders and part of a system of investor-owned hospitals operating several facilities. However, research in the USA indicates that multi-hospital systems may have higher costs than independent hospitals. Owing to the market failures in healthcare arising from factors such as asymmetry of information and uncertainty, competition will not necessarily result in efficient outcomes. The further consolidation of hospitals and the creation of large hospital conglomerates in the 1990s have resulted in the hospital market becoming even more concentrated, thereby reducing the options available to managed care organisations and possibly also raising prices.

Much of the argument for hospital concentration and merger is that by increasing their size, hospitals will achieve lower average costs, exploiting economies of scale. Similarly, unit costs may be reduced by producing different services through the use of common resources for joint production, frequently referred to as economies of scope. Parallel arguments are used in relation to achieving quality gains through the exploitation of economies of scale and scope. In Chapter 3 Aletras Vassilis systematically reviews a wide and complex range of research which has attempted to quantify these economies of scale and scope and estimate the 'optimal' size of hospitals. The literature on economies of scale in the provision of acute hospital services is extensive and covers a wide range of statistical techniques. The methodological quality of published papers varies

widely, as might be expected, but the results appear to be relatively consistent:

- the majority of studies report constant or decreasing returns to scale for acute hospital services in the range of hospital sizes found in the studies. If economies of scale are evident, then these appear to be exploited fully at a relatively low level (in the range of 100–200 beds);
- diseconomies of scale do appear to be a significant feature of hospital production, although it is difficult to generalise the level at which average costs may be expected to begin to rise. A range of 300–600 beds is consistent with the evidence;
- the extent or size of any economies or diseconomies of scale cannot be estimated reliably from the literature.

It is difficult to place these results in a UK context given the lack of standard information available on NHS bed numbers by hospital. A preliminary analysis of the IHSM Health and Social Services Yearbook (1997/98) reveals that in England there are in the region of 246 Trusts categorised as 'acute' or 'acute and community' or 'whole district'. Analysis has been undertaken of the 235 Trusts for which bed numbers are available in the Yearbook, comprising approximately 620 hospital sites (i.e. on average 2–3 sites per Trust; range 1–12 sites). It is clear that hospitals with 300 beds or more (over half of all acute hospitals in England lie in this size category) account for around 80% of the total bed capacity in the NHS in England; in other words, hospital supply is already fairly concentrated and it is not clear that economies of scale may be easily achievable in practice.

An issue of specific interest is whether increasing concentration by, for example, hospital mergers can be expected to generate efficiency gains in the NHS through the exploitation of economies of scale. The literature which deals directly with the gains from merger (mostly from the USA) has not generally shown dramatic improvements in efficiency or expected savings, and this is consistent with the more general research evidence on economies of scale. If, as that evidence suggests, economies are exhausted at low levels, mergers cannot be expected to offer opportunities for improvements in efficiency when the constituent hospitals are already above the threshold level and working efficiently.

This is a conclusion which may appear counter-intuitive. Trust mergers, for example, are expected at least to eliminate duplication and to reduce the costs of administration and management. However this, if it happens at all, is a partial effect. The relevant measure is the change in *total* costs per episode and not (for example) the change in management costs alone. Assuming a hospital is otherwise efficient, the evidence from the literature predicts that as scale is increased, even though management costs may be reduced, average total costs may well remain constant or increase (diseconomies of scale). This could be due to a decline in standards of management leading to reduced efficiency, or to a redistribution of management tasks to non-traditional managers (such as clinicians or nurses), which affects output.

It is important, however, to recognise that the literature on economies of scale is directly relevant only to those hospitals which are technically efficient: that is, operating on the 'efficiency frontier'. All this evidence can tell us is whether a hospital with 250 beds, which was operating efficiently, would have higher or lower unit costs if it expanded to 400 beds and was equally efficient. Evidence that opportunities for reducing costs through economies of scale are insignificant is not in itself a conclusive argument against concentration. Where hospitals are characterised by excess capacity and unused facilities, concentration (or merger) may reduce overall unit costs by taking surplus capacity out of the system. Alternatively, where existing facilities are in need of modernisation or refurbishment, a capital scheme involving the concentration or merger of more than one site may offer the most efficient or feasible solution. In these cases it is not the increase in size or concentration that results in efficiency gains but, for example, the reduction of excess capacity.

Another argument for concentrating hospital provision and for mergers is that improvements in clinical outcomes will follow from increasing the volume of activity at hospital or clinician level or both. Evidence on the relationship between volume and (mostly) hospital mortality rates comes from a large body of international literature which is reviewed by Amanda Sowden and colleagues (Chapter 2). The majority of the more than 200 (mostly observational) studies included in the literature review report a reduction in poor outcomes as volumes increase. However, the apparent strength of this observation may be misleading because of the inadequate handling in many studies of differences in patient case-mix.

Studies of differences in hospital mortality rates need to distinguish between the effects of differences in severity of illness and the effects of differences in quality of care. Higher mortality rates in low-volume hospitals, for example, may be due to differences in case-mix and severity rather than to differences in the skills of clinicians or quality of care. Variations in case-mix have a crucial influence on the interpretation of outcome data from observational studies, and unmeasured differences in patient populations between hospitals or doctors with different volumes of activity may produce misleading results because of the effects of confounding.

The more that patient characteristics are taken into account, for example by statistical adjustment for confounding, the more likely it is that an unbiased assessment of the association between hospital or physician volume and outcomes will be obtained. Routine hospital data rarely provide sufficient detail to adjust adequately for case-mix, and studies which adjust for the risk of death based on detailed prognostic data are the most valid. The majority of the studies identified in the review make no adjustment for differences in the risk factors affecting survival. Even when adjustments are made, it is not clear that variables used in these adjustments (such as age and diagnosis) are sufficiently good predictors of outcome. The importance of adequate adjustment is well illustrated in the statistical analysis of studies of coronary artery bypass graft (CABG) surgery, which shows that the estimated benefit of increasing volumes above 200 procedures a year diminishes the better the quality of the study.

When attention is focused on the better quality studies (those with adequate adjustment for the effects of confounding), the evidence for a relationship between volume and outcome is much less clear, although it is still significant in a number of cases. Two conclusions emerge. First, most of the existing research, because it does not sufficiently take account of differences in case-mix, probably over-estimates the impact of volume of activity on quality of care. Second, because none of the research indicates that increasing activity over time leads to improvements in clinical outcome, it is difficult to infer from the results of those cross-sectional studies which show better outcomes in higher-volume units that similar differences in outcomes can be expected by the expansion of an existing unit. The most that the research evidence can support is a conclusion that if there are significant quality gains from increased volume, these gains appear to be exhausted at relatively low thresholds. Volumes of activity above these thresholds should be achievable in most cases without significant structural change, but may require a more sharply defined internal division of labour between consultant staff (which may be consistent with increased specialisation within disciplines).

It may be that 'clinical systems of care' which are not limited by managerial or physical boundaries may provide a better balance between clinical and cost-effectiveness and accessibility than single facilities with all of the specialist services available in-house. They are likely to be more flexible because the optimum range of population served will vary across client groups and perhaps over time as new technologies develop. The necessary co-ordination of services to produce such collaboration across hospitals and units will require strong strategic direction from regulators and commissioners.

Mergers represent a particular mechanism for the concentration of service delivery. The rationale underlying mergers in the healthcare sector is considered further by Brian Ferguson and Maria Goddard in Chapter 6. Attention is focused particularly on horizontal mergers: that is, mergers between hospitals which provide a similar range of services. The authors point out that in England, where hospitals are already more concentrated than in the USA, several mergers have been approved and have taken place, often as part of reviews of acute service provision. A number of arguments are typically advanced in favour of mergers, such as the removal of excess capacity where genuine over-supply (under-utilisation of fixed resources) exists. A survey of Regional Offices reported in Chapter 6 demonstrates that there is also a strong belief amongst managers in the NHS that mergers will exploit economies of scale and scope, improve the quality and seamlessness of care, and aid the training of specialist staff.

In an overview of the literature on mergers in the healthcare and other sectors in the UK and USA, the authors conclude that many of the anticipated gains from mergers are never realised. Predicted efficiency gains often do not appear and indeed unforeseen costs often arise due to difficulties in integrating systems and personnel from different organisations. In view of this, policies which assume that a process of hospital merger will result in substantial resource savings are possibly over-optimistic. Each case is different and the local context is very important. If mergers are proposed as a solution to perceived service deficiencies, the onus should be on those who advocate change to explain the process by which benefits are to be realised and to evaluate these.

The pressure for concentration of services does not come solely from economic or market forces. The recommendations of the associations of healthcare professionals such as the Royal Colleges and specialist societies can also have an impact on service configuration, an issue discussed by Robin Dowie and Hugh Gravelle in Chapter 5. The service recommendations of Royal Colleges and other professional associations, although not enforceable, nevertheless impact upon the behaviour of healthcare purchasers and may constrain the ability of units not conforming to their guidance to attract high-quality staff. Of particular importance are the requirements of the Royal Colleges and higher training committees for training recognition. These are enforceable and may result in hospitals having staffing problems if training recognition is withheld.

Unfortunately the knowledge base for the development of these recommendations is very poor and there is little evidence of the relationship between length or type of training and skill acquisition and maintenance. As a result the training recommendations are developed on the basis of expert opinion which may have only limited justification. The potential impact of these recommendations on service configuration and levels of specialisation is particularly worrying, especially since there appears to be little cross-college or specialist co-ordination and little discussion with managers about the likely service effects before they are published. The role of the 'generalist', or at least generalist core skills, is something that we may lose to our cost. It appears sensible that colleges should work together to review requirements and recommendations in a consistent fashion. It would also be helpful for such deliberations to be informed by discussions with academics from various disciplines and health service managers responsible for healthcare commissioning and the provision of services.

Within the UK other factors are seen as important forces for increased concentration of hospital services: in particular the reduction in the hours of junior doctors and the reform of specialist medical training are considered to be particularly influential. The Calman reforms, which came into effect from April 1996, are expected to lead to a shorter training period, a reduction in the service contribution of trainees and a long-term reduction in the relative size of the trainee-doctor workforce. Unless training requirements are not rigorously enforced, an implication is that the acquisition of training recognition will become more difficult in small hospitals, in which trainees cannot see an appropriate number and mix of patients in the reduced period available for training.

Against this background, other factors affect the configuration of services, such as the imperative for hospitals to achieve target reductions in management costs, and the more general pressures on Health Authorities and Trusts to reduce the unit costs of health services through efficiency savings. Concentration of services through Trust mergers or service rationalisation has often been seen, possibly mistakenly, as a way of achieving both of these goals.

The implication arising from many of the contributions to this volume is that there is no compelling reason to believe that further concentration of hospital services in general, and mergers in particular, will result in improved efficiency (through exploiting economies of scale) or in automatic improvements in the quality of clinical outcomes. In assessing the potential negative effects of increased concentration on access and utilisation, the implications for disadvantaged groups in particular should not be overlooked. Even where a specific impact on costs, outcomes or utilisation can be demonstrated in the literature, the process by which such effects are generated is poorly understood. One clear policy implication is that the onus to demonstrate that the potential benefits outweigh the costs should be on the parties proposing changes in the pattern of service configuration.

The accounts of two NHS Chief Executives in Chapter 9 have important lessons. Peter Kennedy reminds us that the management of professional relationships and how it impacts on teamwork and the co-ordination of facilities may be more important factors in cost-effectiveness than increasing volume and sub-specialisation. This is echoed by Jane Emminson who warns against purchaser service reviews and argues for better leadership and joint working between all the local players including GPs, service users and Community Health Councils, within an explicit service and financial framework, to find ways of promoting improvements in the quality of care.

CHAPTER CONTENTS

2

Volume of activity and healthcare quality: is there a link?

Amanda J. Sowden, Ian Watt,
Trevor A. Sheldon

2.1 BACKGROUND

In many countries there is a tendency towards the centralisation of hospital services into larger units. Amongst the variety of forces underlying this trend is a widely held belief that hospitals (and clinicians) that carry out higher volumes of a procedure or treat more patients with a condition provide a higher quality of care (Bunker et al, 1982). Managed care organisations in the USA and purchasers in the UK will often look at the size and volume of activity as a proxy for quality and in 'credentialing' clinicians or hospitals. The Medical Royal Colleges and specialist associations in England set volume standards which they believe should provide a minimum threshold for volumes of certain procedures (see Chapter 5).

In the Netherlands some operations have been regionalised by regulation: open heart surgery, for example, can only be performed in licensed hospitals, in which a minimum of 600 procedures must be carried out each year (Banta & Bos, 1991). Similarly, in the United States, the American College of Surgeons recommended that open-heart surgery teams perform at least 150 operations per year (American College of Surgeons, 1984). In a report of the Joint International Society and Federation of Cardiology/ World Health Organisation Task Force on Coronary Angioplasty it was recommended that a physician performing percutaneous transluminal coronary angioplasty should carry out a minimum of about one case per week (American College of Cardiology, 1988).

These recommendations both derive from and reinforce the general impression that doing more results in doing better, even after training is completed. This impression is fuelled by a large body of research from around the world over the last 20 years which has examined the relationship between volume of hospital and/or physician activity and clinical outcomes. A number of reviews of this literature have been published which have also promulgated the consensus (Luft et al, 1979; OTA, 1988; Black, 1990, Banta et al, 1991; Banta et al, 1992; Stiller, 1994; Ministry of Health, 1994).

This issue has policy significance in that costly reconfigurations of services, such as regionalisation and mergers, are taking place, partly fuelled by or at least legitimised by the common sense view that increasing the volume of services will result in quality gains. It is often the case in policy making that strongly held views about what will increase quality or efficiency turn out to have little foundation. Managers implementing the recommendations of management consultants advocating the latest fashions as certain ways of achieving increased performance are often disappointed by the poor outcome. If healthcare policies are to be more 'evidence based' then it is important to examine, comprehensively and critically, the relevant knowledge base. Against this background we carried out a systematic review of the research to assess the extent to which the consensus was supported by reliable research evidence for a volume–outcome relationship.

A systematic review of research involves the systematic identification of relevant research reports and critical appraisal of the studies in order to determine validity (NHS Centre for Reviews and Dissemination, 1996). This approach is now recognised as a reliable and objective approach to assessing the strength of evidence. The three main questions addressed in this review were:

● what is the evidence of a relationship between hospital or physician volume and patient outcomes?
● to what degree are the results common across procedures and conditions?
● to what extent are any reported differences in outcome associated with volume really attributable to volume, or explainable by other factors such as patient case-mix?

The systematic review involved searching MEDLINE, using both key words and Mesh headings (1980–1996), and other electronic databases such as Embase, Health Planning and Administration, Dissertation Abstracts and Entis (Research report database). Medical Care, a key relevant journal, was hand-searched, references of identified studies were checked and experts in the field were contacted to help identify published and unpublished studies.

Full details of the methods used to conduct this review and tables of all the studies included are given elsewhere (NHS Centre for Reviews and Dissemination, 1997).

2.2 HOW MUCH RESEARCH?

A total of 220 evaluations were found which examined the relationship between the volume of healthcare activity and some measure of healthcare outcome. These covered a wide range of clinical procedures, services and diagnoses, including cardio-vascular surgery, respiratory medicine, abdominal procedures, orthopaedic surgery, intensive care, urology/gynaecology, trauma care, AIDS, cataract surgery and cancer.

Research usually takes the form of an analysis of data from one or more years in which the outcomes of patients treated in hospitals with a larger volume are compared with those of patients treated in units performing smaller volumes. Sometimes a volume threshold or cut-off is used to denote high or low volume, such as 100 or 200 procedures per year. Alternatively, studies use regression analysis to see if there is a continuous relationship or trend in volume and outcome. The thresholds used may vary significantly across studies even for the same procedure.

Most of the studies exclusively examined the volume of procedures at the level of the hospital or unit. However, more recently studies have looked at clinician-level volumes or, more rarely, both. The nature of the outcomes measured also varies. Because these data are often routinely collected, researchers have little control over the sorts of information they can use. Outcome data are usually a measure of patient deaths such as the in-hospital or short-term mortality rate.

Most of the research was carried out in the USA principally because a large amount of data are collected routinely as part of administrative databases, as side products of the billing and reimbursement process.

2.3 QUALITY OF THE RESEARCH – ACCOUNTING FOR CASE-MIX

There are problems with using such routine or other observational data to assess the effect of volume on outcome. Most important is the likelihood that the sorts of patients treated in larger units will be different from those admitted to smaller ones. For example, one group may be sicker than another, or have a greater severity of illness or possibly other characteristics that adversely affect outcome such as increased age and coexisting illnesses (co-morbidities). There may also be socio-economic differences in the catchment populations. Differences in the patient outcomes, therefore, rather than being determined only by differences in quality of care related to volume, may instead be a reflection of differences in case-mix. If case-mix is not adequately taken into account, it is impossible to isolate the effects of volume. Instead, variation in mortality due to differences in patients may be mistakenly attributed to volume effects. This problem is referred to as confounding and can limit the interpretation of any sort of non-randomised study (Frater and Sheldon, 1993).

Studies of hospital mortality rates, therefore, need to distinguish between the effects of differences in severity of illness and differences in quality of care. Higher mortality rates in low-volume hospitals, for example, may be due to a higher proportion of emergency or urgent cases, whereas lower mortality rates in high-volume hospitals may reflect the better results obtained from a greater number of elective procedures and a lower-risk patient population. In order to control for the effects of this confounding, studies should collect data on those factors likely to influence outcome, such as patient characteristics and severity of main and accompanying illness, and adjust for any differences in these factors between the patients treated in the different hospitals. The adequacy of this adjustment is likely, therefore, to affect the quality of the study. Systems which adjust for the risk of dying based on detailed clinical data seem to be the most valid.

Each included study was classified in order to assess the adequacy of adjustment of case-mix and thus the validity of the findings. For this, a hierarchy of patient case-mix adjustment was developed. Each of the studies was given a score from 0 to 3 depending on the extent to which adjustment for patient case-mix had been made: the more comprehensive the adjustment the higher the score. Any studies which used a randomised design were given a score of 3. Table 2.1 outlines the scoring system used.

For each relevant study, data were extracted in a systematic way, so as to highlight the type of procedure or condition, the setting, the health professionals involved, the methods used and the results. Studies were grouped according to the procedure or condition, and within this, studies were ranked according to the extent of adjustment for patient case-mix. Patient case-mix adjustment scores were allocated by two reviewers. Overall, under a quarter of the evaluations were thought to have adequately adjusted for case-mix and so were assigned a score of 3.

The importance of adjustment for case-mix on the estimates of the effect of volume on outcome can be illustrated with respect to coronary artery bypass graft surgery. Twenty-four of the identified studies examined the relationship between volume and outcome for coronary artery bypass graft surgery (CABG) for people with heart disease. This was the most studied condition and also shows a wide range in study quality. Six studies were excluded

Table 2.1 Classification for scoring the adequacy of case-mix adjustment

Adjustment score	Criteria
0	no case-mix adjustment
1	adjustment for demographic variables
2	adjustment for demographic variables and comorbidity
3	adjustment for demographic variables, comorbidity and stage or severity of illness

because they duplicated analysis on the same data sources for the same years, leaving 18 non-duplicate studies from the USA which examined data between 1979 and 1996 (Luft et al, 1979; Rosenfeld et al, 1987; Kelly and Hellinger, 1987; Farley & Ozminkowski, 1992; Williams et al, 1991; Burns & Wholey, 1991; Leape et al, 1993; Hannan et al, 1995; Maerki et al, 1986; Showstack et al, 1987; Johnson, 1988; Grumbach et al, 1995; Hannan et al, 1989; Riley & Lubitz, 1985; Hannan et al, 1994; Hughes et al, 1987; Clark, 1996, Shroyer et al, 1996). These studies mainly used the in-hospital mortality rate as their outcome measure and adjustment for patient case-mix ranged from no adjustments to specific clinical risk factors for cardiac surgery.

Data from each individual study were extracted by using the cut-off point closest to 200 procedures per year to define high and low-volume hospitals. This figure was chosen as it was the cut-off point commonly used by the researchers and therefore allowed comparison across studies. Additionally, a number of studies have reported that there is a threshold of around 200 procedures per year. Data from studies in which volume had been analysed as a continuous rather than categorical variable were not included in this pooling as it was not possible to extract the necessary data (Kelly & Hellinger, 1987; Farley & Ozminkowski, 1992; Burns & Wholey, 1991; Hughes et al, 1987; Shroyer et al, 1996). Two other studies were also excluded from the pooling exercise: the outcome assessed in one study was not mortality (Leape et al, 1993) and in the other study all hospitals were high volume (Williams et al, 1991).

The estimates of benefit associated with higher volume for each study were plotted against the case-mix adjustment scores given to each study (see Appendix for a discussion of the statistical methods used). Patient variables that have been shown to be significantly associated with increased mortality include: age, sex, previous heart operations, ejection fraction (heart pumping capacity), diabetes, previous myocardial infarction, dialysis dependence, cardiac catheterisation crash, unstable angina, intractable congestive heart failure, emergency procedure, creatinine (heart enzyme) levels > 168 mmol/l, severe left ventricular disease, pre-operative haematocrit (red blood cell volume) < 0.34, chronic pulmonary (lung) disease, prior vascular surgery, reoperation and mitral valve insufficiency (Hannan et al, 1991; Farley & Ozminkowski, 1992).

In total, ten studies were included in the analysis and the prognostic variables controlled for varied from age and sex to clinical risk factors. The studies differed in the number of hospitals and patients included and in their volume categories. One study presented data on a 20 per cent sample of elderly Medicare beneficiaries and as it was unclear how the volumes of patients related to hospital volumes the results of this study were only included as part of a sensitivity analysis (Riley & Lubitz, 1985).

Most of the studies reported a positive relation between volume and outcome (an odds ratio less than 1). Figure 2.1 shows the estimate of the benefit (odds ratio of mortality) associated with carrying out more than 200 procedures per year compared with less than 200 procedures per year for each study plotted against the four point case-mix adjustment scale. This clearly shows that those studies with more adequate adjustment for case-mix (e.g. score 3) have odds ratios closer to 1 and so lower estimates of the benefit of high volume than those with poor adjustment (e.g. score 0 or 1).

This relationship between the adequacy of adjustment and the estimate of the size of the relationship between volume and outcome of care was shown to be statistically significant (see Table 2.2). Model B shows that the interaction term between volume and the degree of adjustment is significant and greater than one. This means that as the degree of adjustment for case-mix increases the estimate of the advantage of increased volume is significantly reduced. A similar analysis of the relationship between the year of the study and the estimated effect on mortality of hospital volume was not significant.

The importance of case-mix adjustment is further illustrated in cardiovascular conditions. In coronary artery bypass graft surgery, hospitals performing fewer than 100 procedures per year were found to have significantly greater

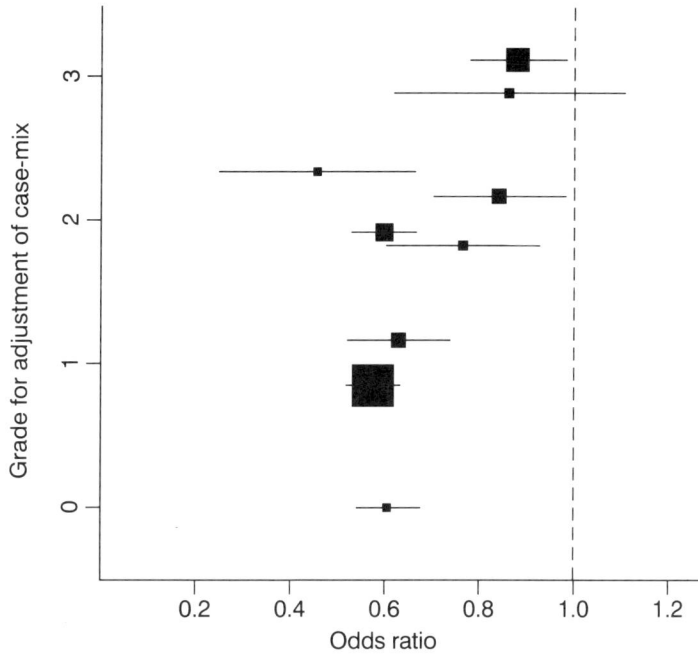

Figure 2.1 How estimates of benefits increased volume (>200) of CABG surgery vary by adequacy of adjustment for case-mix

rates of mortality than hospitals performing more than 100 procedures per year. However, when mortality was risk-adjusted the differences disappeared (Shroyer et al, 1996) Similarly, a study where the outcomes for stroke patients were compared before and after the introduction of a stroke unit found that crude data suggested that patients treated after the introduction of the stroke service were significantly more likely to be alive (Davenport et al, 1996) After adjustment for age and sex this relationship remained significant, however, after adjustment for several prognostic indicators the differences between the two groups were non-significant. This suggested that the improvements found after the introduction of

the stroke service may have been due to differences in case-mix between the two cohorts rather than the new stroke service.

Routine hospital mortality data in the USA (derived from hospital claims forms or patient abstracts) include patients' age, sex, race, principal diagnosis and several secondary diagnoses, the principal procedure and several secondary procedures plus type of admission (emergency or elective). Although researchers tend to use one or more of these administrative variables to adjust for mortality risk, routine claims data provide little relevant information about the patient's condition. Administrative data tend to use fairly simple categories such as whether a disease is or is not present, rather

Table 2.2 Analysis of the relationship between estimates of the effect of volume and the adequacy of the case-mix adjustment

Model	Odds ratio (95% CI)	Statistical significance
Model A Volume	0.66 (0.57, 0.77)	$p < 0.001$
Model B Volume (when adjustment = 0) Adjustment × volume interaction	0.44 (0.36, 0.53) 1.25 (1.14, 1.38)	$p < 0.001$ $p < 0.001$

than the severity of the condition. Clinical data such as the results of physical examinations, laboratory tests or radiological procedures are better predictors of risk. In a review examining the literature on differences in hospital mortality it was reported that out of 16 studies only three used a severity of illness measure to adjust for differences among patients (Fink et al, 1989).

Even in studies using data from clinical databases, which have information on a wider range of relevant factors, one cannot be sure that all the important effects of confounding have been taken into account. In addition it has been shown that validity can be compromised by problems with the accuracy of the data. For example a recent critique of the Cardiac Surgery Reporting System (CSRS), which contains detailed information about all open-heart procedures in New York, has raised questions about the data collection methods. There were significant increases in the prevalence of several risk factors (such as renal failure, low ejection fraction) which were more likely to reflect changes in coding practices than in patients' characteristics. This spurious increase in risk factors accounted for 66 per cent of the increase in predicted mortality and thus for 41 per cent of the total reduction in state-wide risk-adjusted mortality (Green & Wintfeld, 1995).

One study evaluated the volume–outcome relationship between hospitals participating in a randomised controlled trial of angioplasty (Talley et al, 1995). Because people included in trials tend to be more homogeneous than would be expected in observational studies due to of the trial entry criteria, it seems a useful group of patients from which to compare outcomes. Therefore, differences detected between the outcomes of patients treated at different volume hospitals or by different volume surgeons are more likely to be attributable to differences in quality of care rather than to differences in patient case-mix. In this rather small study no statistically significant differences in outcome were detected between people receiving care from an attending physician or a higher-volume 'interventional fellow'. Future research could well benefit from such an approach to evaluation of the volume–outcome relationship.

Another stark illustration of the potential impact of case-mix on estimates of the relationship between volume and quality is provided by a UK study of adult intensive care. One study with grade 3 adjustment for case-mix was based on data derived from the Intensive Care Society's UK APACHE II study and examined the association between the volume of patients admitted to intensive care units and subsequent mortality (Jones & Rowan, 1995). 8,796 patients aged 15 years and above were included from 26 intensive care units in the UK. Average volume levels ranged from 8.3 to 37.7 cases per month. The APACHE II score based on 14 physiologic variables plus weightings for age and chronic ill-health is a validated predictor of mortality in this setting. The score was calculated for each patient. The association which existed between increased monthly volume and reduced mortality using no adjustment disappeared when adjusted using the APACHE II scores

Some volume effects may operate only for sub-groups of patients. Most studies report the results for the whole patient sample, not taking into account any possible differences in the volume effect for different types of patients. This ignores the possibility that the volume effect, if it exists at all, may only operate on sub-groups of patients with particular characteristics, such as baseline risk. It might be the case, for example, that the benefits of being treated in a larger unit, by more experienced clinicians are confined to those patients who have complications or are at high risk of mortality. Patient case-mix can be important therefore in deriving results which are relevant to a practical setting.

Some studies in the perinatal area have examined this issue. For example, one study found that the advantages of Level III hospitals were confined to babies weighing less than 5lb (LeFevre et al, 1992). Another study found that although very low birthweight babies had better survival when born in Level III facilities, normal and low birthweight babies did better when born in Level II hospitals, though case-mix adjustment grade was only 2 in this study (Visisainen et al, 1993). Future research, therefore, needs to look at within-hospital heterogeneity of case-mix.

2.4 OVERALL RESULTS

We have seen that the results of the research examining the relationship between volume and quality are sensitive to their quality of adjustment for the effects of possible differences in case-mix. When attention is focused on the better quality studies (those with adequate adjustment for the effects of confounding) the evidence for a relationship is much less clear, although it is still significant in a number of cases. These results are summarised in Table 2.3.

Two conclusions can be sustained from over 200 evaluations identified. First, most of the existing research, because it does not sufficiently take account of differences in case-mix, probably overestimates the impact of volume of activity on quality of care. Second, because none of the research indicates that increasing activity over time leads to improvements in clinical outcome, it is difficult to infer from the results of cross-sectional studies which show better outcomes in higher-volume units, that similar differences in outcomes can be expected by the expansion of an existing unit.

Table 2.3 Evidence of volume quality relationship from the best quality studies

Procedure/service/ condition	Evidence
Coronary artery bypass graft surgery	• Slightly reduced risk of in-hospital mortality in hospitals carrying out >200 procedures/year (OR = 0.90 95%CI: 0.82-0.98) (see Fig 2.1).
Paediatric heart surgery	• Reduced death rate in hospitals with >300 cases per year compared to hospitals with <10 cases and <300 cases (OR 1/8 and 1/3 respectively).
Acute myocardial infarction	• No significant difference in in-hospital but higher 6-months mortality and lower rate of re-infarction in hospitals with <300 beds (mortality 17% vs 12%). • Significant negative relationship between in-hospital mortality and physician volume (coefficient = –0.05) but not hospital volume.
Cardiac catheterisation	• No physician volume relationship found. Mortality declines by 0.1% for a 100 increase in annual number of hospital procedures (average N of treatments = 400).
Percutaneous transluminal coronary angioplasty	• No significant association between physician volume and angiographic or clinical success. • Reduction in major complications when volume >400/year (OR = 0.66). • No physician volume relationship found for mortality, but more complications, emergency CABG and longer length of stay in physicians carrying out <50 procedures per year.
Abdominal aortic aneurysm	• SMR 30% higher in hospitals with <14 patients/year, but no surgeon relationship found. • 12% mortality for hospitals with <6 procedures compared to 5% in those >38 per year. Double the mortality in low-volume surgeons (<6) compared with high-volume surgeons (>26). • Mortality declines by 1% for an increase of 4 operations per year per hospital (average N of treatments = 23 per year). No evidence of a surgeon volume effect. • 2% increased odds of dying if in hospital with <21 cases compared to >21. This risk difference greater for ruptured aneurysms.
Amputation of lower limb (no trauma)	• SMR 16% higher in hospitals with below-average annual volume (average N of treatments = 10.5).
Gastric surgery	• No significant difference between hospitals with below and above average annual volume (average N of treatments = 24). • Mortality declines by 1% for a 17 increase in the annual number of hospital operations (average N of treatments = 38). No relationship between physician volume and mortality (average N of treatments = 8). • Surgeons carrying out ≤1 procedures annually associated with higher mortality rate than those doing >1. • no relation between physician volume and mortality (average N of treatments = 8)

Cholecystectomy	• SMR 26% higher in hospitals with below-average annual volume (average N of treatments =109). • Hospitals performing <168 procedures a year had a mortality rate of 1.52% compared to 1.21% in those with higher volume. No significant association with surgeon volume found.
Intestinal operations (excluding cancer)	• Hospital mortality higher (8.3%) when <40 operations performed a year than if >40 ops (5.9%). Surgeons with annual volume >8 also associated with lower mortality.
Gall bladder (non-surgical)	• SMR 14% lower in hospitals with below average annual volume (average N of treatments = 73).
Ulcer (non-surgical)	• No statistically significant effect of volume.
Knee replacement	• Higher hospital volume associated with lower risk of complications (average N of treatments = 3.5).
Hip fracture	• No significant effect of hospital volume on mortality (average N of treatments = 45).
Neonatal care	• Infants <28 wks gestation had better survival in intensive care units (>500 days of ventilation/year) compared with special care units (<500 days of ventilation/year). No difference for more mature infants.
Paediatric intensive care	• No statistically significant association found between mortality and monthly volume.
Adult intensive care	• No association between % dying and monthly unit volume.
Prostatectomy	• No statistically significant differences found.
Trauma care	• No statistically significant association between mortality from major trauma and volume across A&E departments with volumes ranging from <10/yr to >90/yr in 3 regions with and without an experimental trauma system (further analysis of data from study by Nichol et al, 1995). • No difference in mortality in a tertiary trauma unit for patients with mainly blunt injuries as it doubled in volume over a 4-year period.
Cataract surgery	• Surgeons carrying out >200 ops per year had greater rate of adverse events (esp. posterior capsular opacification OR = 2.5).
AIDS	• Risk of 30 day mortality was 2.5 times as high when treated in low experience hospitals (<43 patients) than in a hospital having treated >43 patients (RR for 30 day mortality = 2.5).
Breast cancer	• 15% reduction in mortality with surgeons treating >29 new cases/year, but no advantage of >50 compared to >29.
Colon and rectal cancer	• SMR 20% higher in hospitals with below average annual volume (average N of treatments = 17). • No significant association between volume and in-hospital mortality (average N of treatments = 50) or surgeon volume (average N of treatments = 8).
Laparotomy with colorectal resection (for cancer and non-cancer diagnoses)	• No statistically significant differences in mortality or morbidity between surgeons with volumes ranging from 44 to 110 cases per year.
Stomach cancer	• No statistically significant association between mortality and either hospital or surgeon volume.
Malignant teratoma	• 5 year mortality 60% lower in patients treated at a cancer unit which treated over 50% of patients with this cancer in the area.
Oesophageal cancer	• 17% lower rate of operative mortality in surgeons performing >3 ops annually. 4% reduction in 5 year mortality with surgeons treating >5 new cases per year. Most explained by reduced operative deaths.
Pancreatic cancer	• Patients treated by surgeons with highest volume (76 cases in 20 months) had lowest risk of complications (fistula) compared to lower volume surgeons in the same hospital.

* All outcomes in this table are adjusted for case-mix. Results of studies with less adequate adjustment for case-mix (Grade 2 and below) are not summarised here.
OR: Odds Ratio (the ratio of the odds of an adverse event occurring in a higher volume unit compared to a low volume unit; if the OR <1 then there is less risk of a poor outcome in the higher volume unit).
See Effective Health Care 1996 for study details.

2.5 WHY IT IS DIFFICULT TO ASSESS THE VOLUME–QUALITY RELATIONSHIP

The literature on links between volume of activity and clinical outcomes suggests that for some procedures or diagnoses there may be some quality gains as volume increases. In other areas the literature suggests an absence of significant volume gains. Therefore, generalisation is not possible. Other reviews of the literature have reported similar findings and have tended to conclude that the evidence was sufficient to support the concentration of services for some procedures (Banta & Bos, 1991; Office of Technology Assessment, 1988; Ministry of Health, 1994; Luft et al, 1990). In contrast, one recent review examining the outcome of patients with solid cancers found that the literature did not support the idea that centralisation of treatment leads to improved results (Jarhult, 1996). One UK review examining outcomes in patients undergoing surgical procedures was also fairly sceptical about the relationship between volume and outcome and concluded that, even though differences in outcome exist between hospitals, the volume–outcome literature does not prove a causal link (Houghton, 1994).

In the procedures or specialities where volume–quality links have been reported (from the best quality studies) the results are still difficult to interpret for a number of reasons.

2.5.1 Random variation

Outcomes of care are a function not only of patient characteristics and quality of care but also of random events. When outcomes differ between hospitals or clinicians it is important to consider how much of the variation could have occurred by chance. A study where a re-analysis (using more appropriate statistical methods) was performed on computerised discharge data for all adult patients with pneumonia in central Pennsylvania found that variation which was explainable as random had been incorrectly attributed to variations in hospital quality (Localio et al, 1995).

2.5.2 Are the outcomes measured appropriate?

Information on in-patient deaths is readily available in the USA from either hospital discharge abstracts or claims data. However, the use of mortality in these studies is problematic for two reasons. First, the mortality rates recorded usually relate to in-patient deaths only or at best 30-day mortality. This may not be a good proxy for longer-term survival. Indeed differences in short-term survival may simply reflect different discharge policies between hospitals. A hospital that discharges patients at higher risk of dying would as a consequence register a lower in-patient mortality rate. A study by the Stanford Centre for Health Care Research found that a substantial proportion of deaths (for particular conditions) occurred outside the hospital (Staff of the Stanford Centre, 1976).

Second, and more fundamental, mortality over whatever time period can only ever be a partial measure of quality. While it may be the most accessible outcome measure available, it is unlikely to be the most appropriate one. Morbidity and quality of life can be equally important outcomes and increased survival may sometimes be achieved at high cost to the patient. In hip replacement, for example, more appropriate outcome measures are likely to be technical success, morbidity and patient satisfaction, yet in most of the studies reviewed the outcome measured was mortality (Heaton et al, 1995). Health status is more difficult to quantify than mortality and data on quality of life are not routinely collected and recorded. Length of hospital stay is sometimes measured as a proxy for complication rates, as a longer length of stay might be suggestive of post-operative complications, however, this has rarely been validated. Relatively few of the studies reviewed measured outcomes other than mortality, although the studies evaluating outcomes in trauma care tended to focus on avoidable deaths often determined by review of coroners' reports, rather than just mortality rates. Mortality would seem to be particularly inappropriate as an outcome measure for low-risk procedures. To accurately measure quality of care for such procedures more sensitive measures are needed.

The use of effectiveness rates alone for measuring quality have also been questioned. It has been suggested that the appropriate use of a medical procedure also needs to be considered as this is an integral component of the quality of care delivered to patients (Choudhry et al, 1994).

2.5.3 What are high and low volume?

In the majority of studies reviewed volume was measured as the number of patients or procedures per year, although studies have used other periods of time. Some studies have included volume as a continuous measure in a regression analysis to assess whether volume is related to outcome. Others compare the outcome above and below the mean volume for a particular group of hospitals or clinicians, while others choose some threshold or cut-off point to represent high and low volume. In many of the studies where volume is specified as a categorical variable the rationale behind the cut-off points used to define the categories chosen is not clear. What is considered high and low-volume varies enormously between procedures, for example where a hospital performing 50 hip replacements per year might be considered a high-volume facility, a hospital performing 200 CABG operations per year might be considered low volume. Volumes within procedures also vary considerably. In CABG surgery, for example, some studies used above and below 200 procedures per year to define high and low volume while one adopted a cut-off point of 650 procedures per year. These inter-study variations make it very difficult to summarise the research evidence and translate these findings into useful policy recommendations.

2.5.4 Hospital or physician volume?

Research has tended to concentrate on the number of procedures carried out in a hospital rather than on the number performed by each clinician. This is due in part to the lack of data on clinician activity and outcomes and the smaller numbers of events per clinician. Any observed relationship between volume and outcome at the hospital level may in fact be related to the volume or experience of the surgeon carrying out the procedure. Alternatively it may be related to a whole host of variables such as operating-room staff, surgical techniques used, etc. High-volume hospitals were found to be larger, more urban, more expensive, and more likely to be teaching hospitals or affiliated with medical schools.

Some studies have examined the relationship between mortality and physician volume. However, it is not clear whether high-volume physicians work in higher-volume hospitals (or whether the relationship between higher-volume hospitals and mortality is really an effect of having high-volume physicians). In other words the studies which simply use the physician volume variable, alone or with hospital volume, are not able to distinguish between any hospital or physician effects. In order to be able to sensibly consider the potential contribution of each of these effects together and separately the analysis needs to examine the interaction between hospital and physician volume. One study (Hughes et al, 1987) which examined both the hospital volume and the proportion of patients in the hospital operated on by low-volume physicians came close to looking at this. However, no interaction terms were included. This study found that independent of hospital volume, the lower the proportion of patients treated by low-volume physicians, the lower the mortality rate in a number of surgical procedures. Physician volume was not as significantly associated with mortality as was hospital volume. Ideally multilevel modelling techniques should be employed which allow the patient, clinician and hospital-level effects to be analysed appropriately (Rice & Leyland, 1996).

All the physician volume studies are affected by problems with the definition of volume where, for example, the consultant physician may not have been the person who did the operation. Also, it is not clear whether a physician's total experience with other similar operations is taken into account. For example in colorectal cancer surgery the number of similar gastro-intestinal operations performed may affect outcome.

One study assessed hospitals' total experience with heart transplants to determine whether the outcomes in low-volume centres were a function of low volume directly or a function of overall experience. Aggregate outcomes in newly established low-volume centres were compared in their initial year to outcomes in the second year. Mortality rates increased significantly in the second year of operation, suggesting that experience assessed as time doing the operation is not a proxy for volume (Hosenpud et al, 1994).

If a volume–outcome relationship does exist for clinicians it may be that some of the quality gains are due to higher-volume clinicians' keeping up with the literature and the use of the most appropriate management practices available as opposed to their acquisition of purely personal (manual) skills. If this is the case then quality improvement may be achieved in other settings by clinicians with lower volumes adopting guidelines based upon best practice. Thus where outcomes of a procedure are poor there may be a number of measures other than attempts to manipulate volume that could possibly improve results (Hannan et al, 1994).

It is likely that the underlying effects will be the result of a complex interaction between physician and hospital volume and future research should investigate the correlation between hospital and physician volume in order to better understand the nature of any associations.

2.5.5 Direction of causality?

Positive relationships between high volume and outcome could be used to support the 'practice makes perfect' hypothesis. It seems plausible, as higher volume means greater experience with a particular procedure. Alternatively, in some healthcare systems the same results may support a 'selective referral' hypothesis, in which hospitals with good outcomes attract more patients. It may also be the case that higher-volume hospitals attract better clinicians.

The direction of causality is ambiguous since the majority of studies used data from a cross-section of hospitals observed at specific points in time, rather than from a cohort of hospitals over a period of time. Such data are unable to provide the evidence needed to show whether quality would improve if smaller hospitals increased their volume. Changes in volume over time need to be monitored in order to provide such evidence. Only a small number of the studies reviewed used a longitudinal design to assess the effects of changes in volume over time. Where units grew in size over time no improvements were found as hospitals increased their volume even when cross-sectional associations had been found (Boles, 1994; Waddell et al, 1991).

2.5.6 Precise definition of procedure

The procedure whose outcome is being measured should be precisely defined because complication rates for similar procedures may differ. Thus any differences detected in outcome may be due to risks associated with particular procedures rather than to the volume of procedures performed. An example is in total hip replacements, where the outcomes for the two main types (cemented and uncemented) differ. Outcomes for non-cemented prostheses have tended to be poorer than for cemented prostheses (*Effective Health Care*, 1996). Therefore, any comparison in outcomes between hospitals needs to take into account the likely effect of differences in the type of procedure performed.

2.6 CONCLUSIONS AND IMPLICATIONS

Overall, the literature on links between volume of activity and clinical outcomes suggests that for some procedures or specialities there may be some quality gains as hospital or clinician volume increases. In other areas the research suggests an absence of significant volume gains. However, any association found may be confounded by other variables such as differences in patient case-mix between high and low-volume hospitals (or clinicians). The bulk of the research, because it does not sufficiently take into account case-mix differences, probably overestimates the size of the impact of volume on the quality of care. In the few cases where volume–quality links have been suggested by more reliable studies, the thresholds indicated in some studies are relatively low and could be reached through specialisation of tasks within a hospital rather than through an increase in the size of the provider. However, where volume is associated with quality, the direction of causation is not established. It is difficult to use findings of a positive relationship between volume and outcome across hospitals or clinicians to infer what would happen to healthcare outcomes if existing low-volume units expanded.

It is likely that outcomes are dependent upon a combination of factors reflecting hospital, clinician and indeed patient characteristics. Future research needs to move away from simple analysis of statistical linear associations and instead explore the complex range of factors which may influence healthcare outcomes. At present, the emphasis in UK health policy with respect to hospital volume is on centralisation of hospital services, reflecting a number of pressures such as cost, trends in specialisation and training, etc.

Policy to concentrate hospital services in larger units may be driven by a number of considerations. Even if the stated rationale for centralisation of services is to improve outcomes, this may be just a 'fig leaf' for the policy maker to hide behind rather than give more potentially less publicly-acceptable justifications (e.g. cost saving).

However, at least some of the driving force behind proposals to concentrate services is a belief that such moves will improve the quality of care. In spite of this, the influence that this review of the research may have on policy makers is unclear. The overall message from research into the relationship between volume of activity and clinical outcomes is cautious, hedged with uncertainties and may not be strong enough to counterbalance the received wisdom in this area. The main voice countering moves to centralise services is often that of the public which, implicitly at least, seems to place a higher value on access than other dimensions of quality such as the promise of improved clin-

ical outcomes. Recent research evidence from the USA indicates that these concerns may be justified. Adjusted mortality was higher for patients initially admitted to hospitals without on-site cardiac technology and they were less likely to undergo cardiac procedures (Wright et al, 1997). In addition, there is often concern about the impact of centralisation of a service on the quality and viability of services remaining in the peripheral unit.

If research is going to play a more significant role in directing policy in this area, then further studies are needed to answer a number of questions. These include:

- which procedures show a volume effect;
- transferability of skills – if a general surgeon undertakes 500 gall-bladder operations a year and comes across his first appendicectomy in 10 years (as occasionally happens with consultants) are his or her 'general skills' sufficient?
- new procedures and whether there is a stage in their development and implementation after which volume effects decrease;
- hospital vs clinician volume;
- volume thresholds and quality – at both lower and upper levels;
- how long are skills retained (if you do 500 procedures one year, then take a sabbatical do you retain the skills when you return?)
- how far can any volume effect be offset by adequate training and use of clinical practice guidelines?

2.7 APPENDIX: STATISTICAL METHODS USED IN THE MODEL SHOWN IN FIGURE 2.1 AND TABLE 2.2

The estimates of benefit associated with higher volume (odds ratio) for each study is plotted against the degree of adjustment used in the study on the four-point classification scale. A statistical model was used to assess whether there was any systematic change in the estimates of the volume effect as the degree of adjustment for patient case-mix was improved. Logistic regression was used to assess the reported risk of death in high (>200) and low (<200) volume hospitals in each study. A covariate indicating high and low volume was included to estimate the effect of volume on mortality. All models also included a covariate for each study, so that the volume effects were estimated on the basis of within study comparisons (Thompson, 1993).

The model presented in this report included interaction terms which measured the modification of any volume effect related to the year of data collection. It is these interaction terms which are of primary interest in the analysis. The statistical models were fitted to data from the nine studies with the high–low volume cut-off point near 200 cases per year. Overdispersion (residual heterogeneity) was accounted for by appropriate rescaling of standard errors. The significance of the variables was assessed from z-scores calculated as the ratio of the effect sizes to the rescaled standard errors (McCullagh & Nelder, 1983; Baker, 1985).

REFERENCES

American College of Cardiology/American Heart Association Task Force 1988 Guidelines for Percutaneous Transluminal Coronary Angioplasty. JACC; 12:529–545.

American College of Surgeons 1984 Guidelines for Minimal Standards in Cardiac Surgery. American College of Surgeons Bulletin; January:67–69.

Baker R J. 1985 Glim 3.77 Reference Manual. Oxford: Numerical Algorithims Group.

Banta D, Bos M 1991 The Relation between Quantity and Quality with Coronary Artery Bypass Graft (CABG) Surgery. Health Policy;18:1–10.

Banta D H, Engel G L, Schersten T 1992 Volume and Outcome of Organ Transplantation. International Journal of Technology Assessment in Health Care; 8:490–505.

Black N, Johnston A 1990 Volume and Outcome in Hospital Care: Evidence, Explanations and Implications. Health Services Management Research 3:108–114.

Boles M D 1994 A Causal Model of Hospital Volume, Structure and process Indicators and Surgical Outcomes [PhD]. Richmond: Virginia Commonwealth.

Bunker J P, Luft H S, Enthoven A 1982 Should Surgery be Regionalised? Surgical Clinics of North America; 62:657–668.

Burns L R, Wholey D R 1991 The Effects of Patient, Hospital, and Physician Characteristics on Length of Stay and Mortality. Medical Care; 29:251–271.

Choudhry N K, Wright J G, Singer P A 1994 Outcome Rates for Individual Surgeons: Concerns about Accuracy, Completeness and Consequences of Disclosure. Surgery; 115:406–408.

Clark R E 1996 Outcome as a Function of Annual Coronary Artery Bypass Graft Volume. Ann Thorac Surg; 61:21–26.

Davenport R J, Dennis M S, Warlow C P 1996 Effect of Correcting Outcome Data for Case-Mix: An Example from Stroke Medicine. BMJ; 312:1503–1505.

Effective Health Care 1996 Total Hip Replacement. Effective Health Care; 2(7).

Effective Health Care 1996 Volume and Health Care Outcomes, Costs and Patient Access. Effective Health Care; 2 (8).

Farley D E, Ozminkowski R J 1992 Volume–Outcome Relationships and Inhospital Mortality: The Effect of Changes in Volume over Time. Medical Care; 30:77–94.

Fink A, Yano E M, Brook R H 1989 The Condition of the Literature on Differences in Hospital Mortality. Medical Care; 27:315–336.

Frater A, Sheldon T A 1993 The Outcomes Movement in the US and UK. In: Drummond M, Maynard A. (eds) Purchasing and Providing Cost-Effective Health Care. Edinburgh: Churchill Livingstone, ch 4:49–65.

Green J, Wintfeld N 1995 Report Cards on Cardiac Surgeons. Assessing New York State's Approach. NEJM; 332:1229–1232.

Grumbach K, Anderson G M, Luft H S, Roos L L, Brook R 1995 Regionalization of Cardiac Surgery in the United States and Canada. JAMA; 274:1282–1288.

Hannan E L, Kilburn H, Bernard H, O'Donnell J F, Lukacik G, Shields E P 1991 Coronary Artery Bypass Surgery: The Relationship Between Inhospital Mortality Rate and Surgical Volume after Controlling for Clinical Risk Factors. Medical Care; 29:1094–1107.

Hannan E L, Kilburn H, Racz M, Shields E, Chassin M R 1994 Improving the Outcomes of Coronary Artery Bypass Surgery in New York State. JAMA; 271:761–766.

Hannan E L, O'Donnel J F, Kilburn H, Bernard H R, Yazici A 1989 Investigation of the Relationship Between Volume and Mortality for Surgical Procedures Performed in New York State Hospitals. JAMA; 262:503-510.

Hannan E L, Siu A L, Kumar D, Kilburn H, Chassin M R 1995 The Decline in Coronary Artery Bypass Graft Surgery Mortality in New York State. JAMA; 273:209–213.

Heaton J, Williams M, Long A, Dixon P, Brettle A 1995 Measuring the Health Outcomes of Total Hip Replacement Through the Commissioning Process. Outcome Measurement Reviews. No 1. Leeds: UK Clearing House for Health Outcomes, May 1995.

Hosenpud J D, Breen T J, Edwards E B, Daily O P, Hunsicker L G 1994 The Effect of Transplant Centre Volume on Cardiac Transplant Outcome. JAMA; 271:1844–1849.

Houghton A 1994 Variation in Outcome of Surgical Procedures. British Journal of Surgery; 81:653–660.

Hughes R G, Hunt S S, Luft H S 1987 Effect of Surgeon Volume and Hospital Volume on Quality of Care in Hospitals. Medical Care; 25:339–358.

Jarhult J 1996 The Importance of Volume for Outcome in Cancer Surgery – an Overview. European Journal of Surgical Oncology; 22:205–215.

Johnson A N 1988 The Relationship between Volume, Quality and Outcome in Hospital Care Delivery [PhD]. Minnesota: Minnesota.

Jones J, Rowan K 1995 Is there a Relationship between the Volume of Work Carried Out in Intensive Care and its Outcome? International Journal of Technology Assessment in Health Care; 11:762–769.

Kelly J V, Hellinger F J 1987 Heart Disease and Hospital Deaths: An Empirical Study. Health Services Research; 22:369–395.

Leape L L, Hilborne L H, Park R E, et al 1993 The Appropriateness of Use of Coronary Artery Bypass Graft Surgery in New York State. JAMA; 269:753–760.

LeFevre M, Sanner L, Anderson S, Tsutakawa R 1992 The Relationship between Neonatal Mortality and Hospital Level. The Journal of Family Practice; 35:259–264.

Localio A R, Hamory B H, Sharp T J, Weaver S L, TenHave T R, Landis J R 1995 Comparing Hospital Mortality in Adult Patients with Pneumonia. A Case Study of Statistical Methods in a Managed Care Programme. Ann Intern Med; 122:125–132.

Luft H S, Bunker J P, Enthoven A C 1979 Should Operations be Regionalised? The Empirical Relationship between Surgical Volume and Mortality. NEJM; 301:1364–1369.

Luft H S, Garnick D W, Mark D H, McPhee S J 1990 Hospital Volume, Physician Volume and Patient Outcomes. Assessing the Evidence. Michigan: Health Administration Press.

Maerki S C, Luft H S, Hunt S S 1986 Selecting Categories of Patients for Regionalization. Medical Care; 24:148–158.

McCullagh P, Nelder J A 1983. Generalised Linear Models. London: Chapman and Hall.

Ministry of Health 1994 Tertiary Services Review: The Final Report. Wellington, New Zealand: Ministry of Health.

NHS Centre for Reviews and Dissemination 1997 Concentration and Choice in the Provision of Hospital Services. The Relationship between Hospital Volume and Quality of Health Outcomes. CRD Report No 8, part I, University of York.

NHS Centre for Reviews and Dissemination 1996 Undertaking Systematic Reviews of Research on Effectiveness: CRD Guidelines for Those Carrying Out or Commissioning Reviews. CRD Report No 4, University of York.

Nichol J, Turner J, Dixon S 1995 The Cost-effectiveness of the Regional Trauma System in the North West Midlands. University of Sheffield

Office of Technology Assessment 1988 The Quality of Medical Care: Information for Consumers. Washington DC: United States Government Printing Office.

Rice N, Leyland A 1996 Multilevel Models: Applications to Health Data. J Health Serv Res Policy; 1:154–164.

Riley G, Lubitz J 1985. Outcomes of Surgery Among the Medicare Aged: Surgical Volume and Mortality. Health Care Financing Review; 7:37–47.

Rosenfeld K, Luft H S, Garnick D W, McPhee S J 1987 Changes in Patient Characteristics and Surgical Outcomes for Coronary Artery Bypass Surgery 1972–82. American Journal of Public Health; 77:498–500.

Showstack J A, Rosenfeld K E, Garnick D W, Luft H S, Schaffazrick R W, Fowles J 1987 Association of Volume with Outcome of Coronary Artery Bypass Graft Surgery, Scheduled vs Non-Scheduled Operations. JAMA; 257:785–789.

Shroyer A L W, Marshall G, Warner B A, et al 1996 No Continuous Relationship Between Veterans Affairs Hospital Coronary Artery Bypass Grafting Surgical Volume and Operative Mortality. Ann Thorac Surg; 61:17–20.

Staff of the Stanford Centre for Health Care Research 1976 Comparison of Hospitals with Regard to Outcomes of Surgery. Health Services Research; 11:112–127.

Stiller C A 1994. Centralised Treatment, Entry to Trials and Survival. Br J Cancer; 70:352–362.

Talley J D, Mauldin P D, Leesar M A, Becker E R 1995 A Prospective Randomised Trial of 0.010 Versus 0.014 Balloon PTCA Systems and Interventional Fellow Versus Attending Physician as Primary Operator in Elective PTCA: Economic, Technical and Clinical End Points. Journal of Interventional Cardiology; 8:623–632.

Thompson S G 1993. Controversies in Meta-Analysis: The Case of Trials of Serum Cholesterol Reduction. Statistical Methods in Medical Research; 2:173–192.

Visisainen K, Gissler M, Hemminki E 1993 Birth Outcomes by Level of Obstetric Care in Finland: a Catchment Area Based Analysis. Journal of Epidemiology and Community Health; 48:400–405.

Waddell T K, Kalman P G, Goodman S J L, Girotti M J 1991 Is Outcome Worse in a Small Volume Canadian Trauma Centre? The Journal of Trauma; 31:958–961.

Williams S V, Nash D B, Goldfarb N 1991 Differences in Mortality from Coronary Artery Bypass Graft Surgery at Five Teaching Hospitals. JAMA; 266:810–815.

Wright S T, Daley J, Peterson E D and Thibault G E 1997 Outcomes of Acute Myocardial Infarction in the Department of Veterans Affairs: Does Regionalisation of Health Care Work? Medical Care; 35: 128–141.

3

Economies of scale and scope

Vassilis Aletras, Andrew Jones, Trevor A. Sheldon

3.1 BACKGROUND

Healthcare costs are rising over time, exacerbating the need to find ways of containing costs, including methods of enhancing efficiency. An important aspect of efficiency is the optimal scale and scope of hospital production. It is often assumed that by concentrating hospital services into larger units, efficiency will be improved because of the operation of economies of scale. Economies of scale refers to a situation in which long-run average costs fall as the scale or volume of activity rises and fixed costs are spread over greater levels of activity, the long-run being a period sufficiently long to permit *all* inputs (even the number of beds) to be variable. Economies are expected in a production process in which fixed costs are high relative to the variable costs of production. Economic theory often assumes a U-shaped relationship between average costs and hospital size. As facility size (and output) increases average costs are thought to decrease (economies). However, increasing scale often implies additional sources of cost, and beyond some critical volume long-run average costs are expected to begin to rise (diseconomies of scale) (Figure 3.1).

Suppose that local demand can be served by one large general hospital or two smaller ones. If economies of scale exist a government agency may choose the former option. In reality, of course, other policy parameters – such as the costs of travelling and delayed emergency treatment – should also be taken into account. Similarly, the presence of economies of scope between hospital services due to cost savings from an increase in the scope (or variety) or joint production of services which a hospital is offering will define the sets of services that should be collected together and operated within the same hospital unit. If, for instance, such savings exist for in-patient and out-patient care, an agency must direct resources towards the development of hospitals which provide both services rather than operate separate entities.

Various sources of scale economies have been suggested. First, a larger scale of operation permits greater opportunities for the division of labour and hence specialisation. Second, there are technological factors giving rise to scale advantages. One such factor is the existence of an initial 'lump' of fixed costs which implies that the unit costs can be reduced with increased production. Another potential technical economy results when a hospital can double the capacity of its buildings by less than doubling the construction costs. Third, there are economies on reserves of labour or materials available to a larger institution, if there is a variable demand for its services. A larger facility is required to keep a smaller proportion of its beds in reserve to meet an unexpected demand. Finally, there may be pecuniary economies, that is quantity discounts and lower interest rates on borrowed capital, enjoyed by larger organisations.

New concepts have been introduced to deal with complex institutions like hospitals which produce a range of different outputs. Ray economies of scale refer to the response of total cost to a proportional change in *all* output categories, keeping other cost determinants constant. However, it may be that scale advantages exist for some services and not for others. Product-specific economies of scale refer to cost changes when provision of a particular service is increased, keeping all other service levels constant.

Economies of scope may result, for instance, from the avoidance of duplication of medical equipment, or from the existence of related clinical specialities on site. Diseconomies of scope may also arise, for example, from an excessive use of expensive medical equipment, unavailable to some members of the medical staff prior to the bundling of the services.

Although the theoretical arguments are strongly in favour of the existence of economies of scale at least up to some level of operation, this needs to be empirically validated. Research on economies of scope is also needed to determine the optimal config-

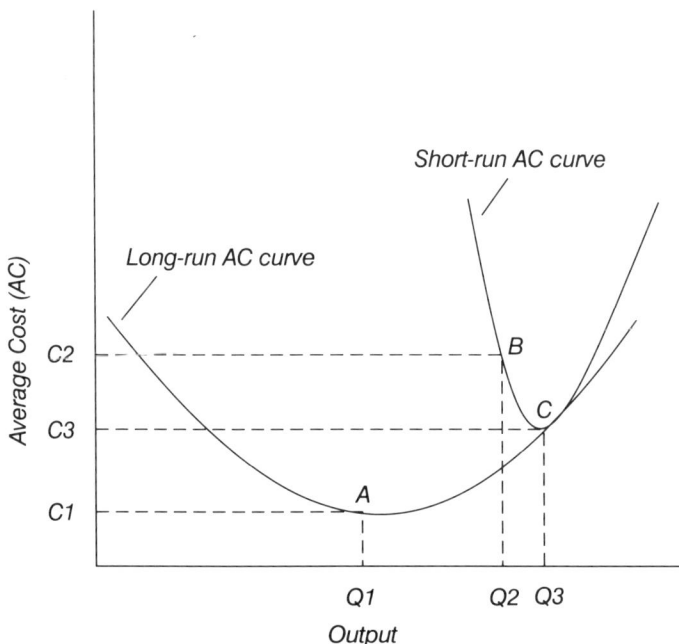

Figure 3.1 Short-run vs long-run cost minimisation in a single-product firm.

uration of service bundles within hospitals. This chapter summarises the results of the research evidence based on a systematic review of the literature carried out using the explicit and structured approach now expected in the field of clinical epidemiology (NHS Centre for Reviews and Dissemination, 1996). The expectation is that a systematic review will provide more valid conclusions based on the overall – rather than piecemeal – evidence via the use of appropriate quality criteria. The methods used are described in detail elsewhere (NHS Centre for Reviews and Dissemination, 1997).

Approximately 100 studies were identified which provided evidence on the existence of economies of scale and scope in the hospital setting. These use a variety of different techniques to assess the existence of economies. Econometric studies, for example, use regression analysis to explore the effects of a number of variables on the average cost of hospital treatment. Other approaches used include data envelopment analysis (DEA), market survival methods and before–after studies looking at the effects of multi-hospital arrangements (e.g. mergers).

As part of the review, the quality of each study was assessed using a set of methodological criteria by which to judge the quality of the studies. Some of the validity criteria were common across studies such as correction for differences in patient case-mix and quality of care between hospitals and over time. Other criteria were specific to the technique being used (see Appendix). When analysing the average costs of hospital output, for example, most studies use either the cost per hospitalised case (or episode) or the cost per patient day. Costs of a hospital admission are not spread evenly because the treatment costs tend to be loaded early on in the stay. Therefore, hospitals increasing efficiency by reducing the average length of stay would appear to be less efficient because the cost per day would increase. Cost per case studies are therefore preferred to those using cost per day. Sections 3.2 to 3.8 summarise the results from different types of studies; details of individual studies are presented elsewhere (NHS Centre for Reviews and Dissemination, 1997). A summary and discussion of the implications is provided in Section 3.9.

3.2 AD HOC COST STUDIES

Studies conducted mainly prior to the mid-1980s have been characterised as 'ad hoc' primarily due to their indiscriminate use of any variable that was thought to be influencing costs and the exclusion of theoretically important structural variables (e.g. input prices).

Thirty-six ad hoc studies were identified but half were excluded because they used the patient day as the unit of output (criterion 1), the service-mix approach alone (criterion 3), or the 'no adjustment approach' over time or across hospitals of Lave and Lave, and Wagstaff (his stochastic model). The remaining studies are based on either the case-mix approach or a combined case-mix/service-mix adjustment, the service-mix presumably standing proxy for the quality of output or technological sophistication.

Almost all of these eighteen studies indicate constant returns or diseconomies. With the exception of Butler's (1995) mixed results, the five studies which adjust better for case-mix indicate constant returns or diseconomies. Finally, Pauly (1978) corrects for case-mix differences by means of an index but also for non-physician input prices by inserting four variables (criterion 5) and simultaneously employs the superior Cobb–Douglas functional form (criterion 2) and reports constant returns.

The finding of constant returns or diseconomies of scale could have been due to the inclusion of large-sized hospitals. However, Feldstein and Schuttinga (1977) and Pauly (1978) report a mean bed size of 180 beds and find constant returns. Evans and Walker (1972) utilise a sample of hospitals of various sizes including very small (<25 beds) and very large (>1,000) and find moderate diseconomies. Economies are only reported for hospitals with fewer than 100 beds. Bays (1980) reports evidence of constant returns for rather small sample hospitals (mean bed size is 124). The exclusion of the physician input price by most of these reinforces the view that economies of scale are absent.

The conclusion from these studies that there are few examples of economies of scale should, however, be treated with caution. First, economies of scale due to the stochastic demand for hospital services are not accounted for in these studies (criterion 6), there might still be uncontrolled case-mix variations (criterion 3), the quality effect has not been dealt with adequately (criterion 7), and computed estimates may not measure true long-run economies (criterion 4). In addition, there may be biases from the use of overly restrictive functional forms and it is not clear which, if any, of the behavioural variables are indeed relevant (criterion 8).

3.3 FLEXIBLE COST STUDIES

Flexible functional forms are used in an attempt to avoid some of the problems associated with the more restrictive ad hoc cost studies. The most common flexible form is the transcendental logarithmic (translog) or a version called the generalised (or hybrid) translog. There are advantages and disadvantages in using flexible functional forms for multiproduct analysis. On the one hand, they typically satisfy – in the empirically estimated region – the theoretical conditions associated with a well-behaved cost function. Moreover, they allow for flexibility in that they do not prejudge the existence or degree of economies of scale and scope and can accommodate product-specific economies of scale and economies of scope.

This increased flexibility, however, is obtained at the cost of greatly reduced parsimony: with just 5 inputs and outputs, 55 parameters would have to be estimated in an ordinary translog model. This is a major limitation in healthcare since controlling for the extreme variation between hospitals in the types of output requires a large number of case-mix and other (e.g. teaching) variables. Another weakness is the potential inability of these functions to provide accurate estimates away from the point at which the function is being approximated – typically the sample means.

After excluding the studies which compute short-run measures (criterion 4), 13 studies remain which report evidence on overall (long-run) economies of scale. Most studies found that the average hospital in the samples used operates under diseconomies or constant returns. Exceptions are the attempts by Burns (1982), Banks (1993), Sinay (1994) and Gaynor and Anderson (1995), which document unexploited economies or report mixed evidence. However, only the studies by Eakin and Kniesner (1988), Vita (1990), Pangilinan (1991), Kemere (1992), Gaynor and Anderson (1995) and Scuffham, et al (1996) employ the hospitalised case as the unit of measurement of hospital output (criterion 1). Hence only the study by Gaynor and Anderson (1995) seems to yield acceptable evidence of economies, though this could well be due to the poor adjustment for input prices and outputs in that study (criteria 5). This is corroborated by the absence of significant economies due to the stochastic demand witnessed by Mulligan (1987). The studies by Burns (1982) and Banks (1993) which document economies can also be criticised on other grounds. Their models fail to meet the regularity conditions (criterion 10) even at the means of the variables. In contrast these conditions are satisfied at the means and even away from the means in the studies by Eakin and Kniesner (1988) and Kemere (1992), which report large diseconomies and constant returns respectively. This work also performs satisfactorily with respect to the cost-minimisation hypothesis (criterion 9). Moreover, Eakin and Kniesner (1988) incorporate a proxy for the physician price, the implication being that Kemere's (1992) model could also be indicative of diseconomies if that price was not omitted (criterion 5).

The interpretation of these results depends on the average size of the hospitals included in the samples. Scuffham, et al (1996) find constant returns for an average hospital of only 125 beds. We argued earlier that the results of this study might be more reliable. However, if it incorporates very different hospital types, ranging from general hospitals to maternity and psychiatric. It may not be legitimate to do this since the underlying production structures might be different. Other studies have also lumped together diverse hospital types (e.g. for- and not-for-profit, teaching and non-teaching) but have at least confined themselves to general hospitals.

The study by Eakin and Kniesner (1988) does not report the mean sizes whereas that by Kemere (1992) documents constant returns for a hospital with a size of about 300 beds and a volume of some 12,500 in-patient discharges and 17,200 out-patient visits. This work also confines the sample to a single state in order to avoid biases from uncontrolled differences in the regulatory environment. Given an over-investment in capital in the hospital industry in the USA the *true* optimum sought in a regulatory regime consistent with long-run cost minimisation may be higher.

Other studies which also perform quite satisfactorily with respect to the validity criteria found diseconomies for smaller average hospitals. Vita (1990), for instance, documents slight diseconomies for an average hospital of 180 beds (about 7,800 inpatient discharges and 30,300 outpatient visits). This might mean that economies are exhausted at even lower size levels than the study by Kemere (1992) indicates. Despite the inability of these studies to pinpoint an exact optimal hospital size there is broad agreement between the more reliable studies that if any economies exist they are quickly exhausted. That is, they might be present only for small hospitals with fewer than 100–200 beds.

Global measures of output-specific economies of scale and economies of scope probably cannot be trusted and might mislead policy makers since the cost functions were not shown to be regular away from the sample means (criterion 10). Local measures of weak cost complementarities, in general, did not support the existence of economies of scope for the average hospital in the long-run at the levels of output aggregation used. This does not rule out the existence of long-run economies of scope; we simply cannot prove their existence. Gruca and Nath (1994) found economies only between general medical (acute) and obstetrics care. Sinay (1994) showed that in one merger episode there were economies prior to the merger between acute and sub-acute care, providing reasons for the consolidations. He did not find any economies in a second episode,

further suggesting that they may be more likely where there is excess capacity. Nevertheless, one limitation of these two studies is the use of the patient day as the unit of measurement of hospital output (criterion 1).

Economies of scope were also not detected by Rozec (1988) who constructed triplets of costs from a hospital without a psychiatric unit, a psychiatric hospital, and a hospital with a psychiatric unit. Hospitals were matched for ownership, length of stay, location and size. However, the absence of scope effects may have been due to the poor matching (e.g. for case-mix).

3.4 ECONOMETRIC PRODUCTION FUNCTION STUDIES

If hospitals minimise costs then information on economies of scale can be retrieved from either the cost function (Sections 3.2 and 3.3 above) or the underlying production function, which describes the relationship between inputs and outputs in physical units. There are only a few reported production studies. The quality of individual production studies was assessed using similar criteria to the ones used for the assessment of cost models.

Mildly decreasing returns to scale were found using three models (Cobb–Douglas, a mixed Leontief–Cobb–Douglas and a more general *ad hoc* production model) in which output is standardised (Feldstein, 1967). A similar result was found in a UK study of *maternity* hospitals using Cobb–Douglas and flexible log-quadratic forms (Lavers and Whynes, 1978). A study of Newfoundland's *cottage* hospitals (mean bed size 29), however, using the same approach, found increasing returns to scale (Brown, 1980).

More reliable estimates were provided by two flexible models. Van Montfort (1981), employing a translog functional form, and using weighted admissions as the dependent variable, found constant returns to scale and positive marginal products for all inputs. Jensen and Morrisey (1986) estimate a production function and find it to be well-behaved in the sense that marginal products for all inputs are positive and decreasing. Using the estimates from their translog model and the sample mean values of the inputs to compute the output elasticities, their sums for the non-teaching and teaching sub-samples are 0.858 and 0.952, both below unity, indicating decreasing returns for the average hospital.

The only included study to find significantly increasing returns in larger hospitals examined 142 New York State hospitals over 1981–1987 (Pangilinan, 1991). However, several important inputs (such as physicians) are omitted and so a Ramsey RESET test indicates that the model is mis-specified.

Despite the apparent consensus that returns to scale are at best constant, caution is warranted as the case-mix problem is treated less satisfactorily than in cost studies and because of the significant multicollinearity that exists between input variables. Moreover, quality differences are ignored and the mean levels of hospital size are rarely reported. However, despite these reservations, the consistency of the results with those of cost analyses is encouraging.

3.5 DATA ENVELOPMENT ANALYSES

In Data Envelopment Analysis a hospital is said to be *relatively* efficient if, in comparison with other hospitals, there is no proof that it utilises any of its inputs inefficiently. The technique constructs empirically, from the observed input/output relations of existing hospitals, what has been known as a 'best practice frontier', which consists of efficient hospitals having the highest total factor productivity in the sample. The relative inefficiency of the remaining ones is given by their position relative to the frontier. The technique is non-parametric, thus imposing only weak assumptions. DEA can readily handle multiple inputs and outputs and has therefore been seen as a useful tool for assessing pure technical or allocative inefficiencies in hospitals. Variable Returns to Scale (VRS) models have been developed which allow identification of whether a particular hospital exhibits increasing, decreasing or constant returns. Banker (1984) also proposed the calculation of the most productive scale size

(mpss) of hospitals, i.e. the point of hospital production at which decreasing returns have not yet started to operate.

Several criteria presented previously for the evaluation of econometric studies – the unit of measurement of hospital output, the adjustment for differences in outputs (e.g. case-mix, teaching), inputs, quality of care, and reservation quality – can also be applied here (see Appendix). An additional criterion is also needed which relates to the success with which an individual study remedies problems regarding the choice of variables and errors in the data which are common in health-service studies.

There is general agreement between studies that hospitals with fewer than 200 and more than 620 beds are scale inefficient, owing to increasing and decreasing returns respectively. However, the evidence is conflicting regarding the precise position of the optimum. Banker et al (1986) and Byrnes and Valdmanis (1994) calculate a mean mpss of 220–260 beds, which does not seem to be in wide disagreement with the position of the optimum that may be inferred from the work of Valdmanis (1992). In the latter, the mean scale efficiency is found to be 0.97–1.00 for public hospitals which have a mean bed size of 350, and 0.92–0.97 for private not-for-profit ones whose mean size is 428.

Maindiratta (1990) examines not only whether input savings might be realised by a hospital, given its observed task, but also whether additional savings could result if the task itself were to be optimally apportioned to a number of smaller hospitals. The findings suggest that decreasing returns set in very gradually so that a hospital must be a lot bigger than its mpss before it pays to apportion its task to smaller units. The largest-size efficient scale exceeds the mpss in some selected hospitals by a factor of 1.55–1.81. The French study by Dervaux et al (1994) suggests that scale efficiency is achieved at 500–620 beds.

Quality of care has not been controlled for adequately, nevertheless, some adjustment has been made in three of the studies. They limited their samples to a particular ownership type (Dervaux et al, 1994; Byrnes and Valdmanis,

1994), or ran different DEA programs for different ownership types (Valdmanis, 1992). In fact, Valdmanis (1992) excluded small and rural, and Byrnes and Valdmanis (1994) teaching hospitals, in order to control further for environmental differences. The other two studies (Banker et al, 1986; Maindiratta, 1990) do not report the types of hospitals included. In addition, all US studies employ data from a single state to control for regulatory differences.

These restrictions may have helped increase the similarity of case-mix between the hospitals. Studies have also directly controlled – to varying degrees – for output heterogeneity. Two research attempts (Banker et al, 1986; Byrnes and Valdmanis, 1994) relied on the use of two to three output variables defined in terms either of patients' age or of type of treatment. Their findings are similar: an optimum well below 400 beds which is insensitive to slight changes in the input/output variables used.

The study by Dervaux et al (1994) suggests higher optimum values of around 500–520, which rises to 620 when case-mix complexity and other activity variables are added. However, these results were not subjected to a sensitivity analysis so they may not be as reliable (criterion 11).

Summing up, there is evidence that the optimum is located in the 220–620 bed region. Evidence from DEA simply indicates that small and very large hospitals may be sub-optimal. Nevertheless, the results of DEA studies should be interpreted with caution. First, differences in quality of care (and presumably case-mix) are inadequately controlled for; second, reservation quality services provided by hospitals in response to demand uncertainty have not been taken into account; finally, sensitivity analysis to examine the potential effects of specification, measurement and sampling errors is not carried out in most studies and not very satisfactorily in the work of Valdmanis (1992).

3.6 SURVIVAL ANALYSES

An alternative approach, survival analysis, shifts attention away from cost and its determinants towards the study of changes in hospital-size distribution over time. It assumes that competition among hospitals of different sizes will bring about the disappearance of hospitals with inefficient sizes. So, rather than trying to directly estimate production functions, it infers the optimal size from the results of the operation of the healthcare market. Hospitals are classified into size classes and the market share of each class over time is recorded. If the market share of a given size class increases over time it is inferred that this is the optimal size. Moreover, hospitals within a class are more efficient (inefficient) the more sharp is the rise (decline) of their share. The technique is to some extent valid in markets other than the purely competitive since oligopolistic firms also have an incentive to adjust to more efficient sizes in search of larger profits.

A heroic further step is to attribute expansion (shrinking) of a size class over time to the presence of economies (diseconomies) of scale. 'Those size categories which grow relative to the rest are presumed to have *some* [emphasis added] advantage over other sizes' (Bays, 1986).

The main problem of interpreting changes in market share is that several factors influence hospital survival, closure and growth. Observed survival and growth of larger hospitals may be due to the exploitation of suppliers or predatory policies. A fall in their market share may be caused by the fear of anti-trust legislation, and the growth of small hospitals may be an attempt to escape anti-trust laws. The size advantage may not be due to scale economies; growth may be partly or wholly ascribed to other factors and the survival approach does not disentangle the portion of growth that can be ascribed to scale economies. Evidence that small hospitals are more likely to fail, for example, does not necessarily support the existence of economies, since smaller hospitals are typically rural hospitals so that location could equally explain the findings.

In principle, nevertheless, progress can be made if some of these other determinants of growth are controlled for. The survival approach implicitly assumes that the magnitude of economies of scale will be large enough to significantly affect the survival of the hospital. This may not be true, so a finding of no significant association between size and hospital survival cannot rule out its existence.

In the context of survival-type analysis, which is an indirect method of studying economies, determining a detailed set of criteria to assess biases from the omission of relevant individual variables is more difficult. However, multi-variate survival analyses which at least control for some potential confounding factors are more reliable than univariate ones. Traditional (univariate) survival methodology has been applied in the hospital setting by Bays (1986), Mobley (1990), Vita et al (1991), and Mobley and Frech (1994).

A more sophisticated approach which controls for other demand-related determinants of survival and growth in order to isolate the size effect was applied to 1980–1989 California hospital data, a period of increased competition and deregulation (Mobley and Frech, 1994). Scale economies in quantity and quality are found to exist jointly up to a point of 325 beds. Similar multi-variate continuous and binary growth/survival models used by Mobley (1990) and Frech and Mobley (1995) found economies of scale to exist up to about 300 beds and an optimum of 200 beds, with a 95 per cent confidence interval extending the range to 370 but with low explanatory power.

Two other studies use logistic regressions to adjust for factors affecting the risk of closure, such as utilisation and market characteristics. Among their differences is the inclusion of a case-mix index by Lillie-Blanton et al (1992) and a DEA efficiency measure by Lynch and Ozcan (1994) as independent variables. The former study finds that hospitals with more than 200 beds are 2.5 times less likely to fail than those with 100–199 beds, and 5 times fewer likely to close than hospitals with fewer than 100 beds. Because it combines all hospitals with more than 200 beds into a single category, it can only be inferred that the optimum lies somewhere in the 200+ region. The study by Lynch and Ozcan (1994) is even less informative in this respect since it uses a single variable for size, which simply indicates that there are economies of scale for larger hospitals. There is a general agreement among these studies that hospitals with fewer than 200 beds are scale-inefficient. The studies by Mobley and Frech (1994) and Frech and Mobley (1995) suggest an optimum of 325 and 200–370 beds respectively, and Mobley (1990) in addition argues that no diseconomies ever set in for larger hospitals.

Simpson (1995) criticises previous studies which claim that sub-100 bed hospitals are inefficient because they utilise California data from periods prior to 1987 when Certificate of Need (CON) legislation was still in effect. Hence the documented decline in market share may have reflected entry restrictions preventing the replacement of the exiting sub-100 bed hospitals by new ones of the same size. Post-1987 hospital data show a large number of sub-100-bed hospitals entering the market.

The results from survival studies cannot readily be interpreted as due to economies of scale and should be interpreted with extreme caution. The low adjusted R^2 (unsatisfactory values of a measure of goodness-of-fit) in the regressions confirms that a large proportion of the variance is unexplained indicating that the effects of many uncontrolled variables possibly correlated with the size variables may exist.

3.7 STUDIES EXAMINING A HOSPITAL SERVICE IN ISOLATION

Thirteen studies which focus on a particular hospital ward or service were identified. These assume that hospital production can be broken down into many independent production procedures, each referring to a particular ward or service. A separate cost or production function can be employed to study the existence and magnitude of scale effects of each service or ward. Since the output produced in these cases is considerably less varied the case-mix problem may be reduced. The studies have used various statistical or econometric techniques.

Some of the validity criteria already developed can be applied here (see Appendix). Moreover, it is crucial to check whether a particular study design does in fact produce estimates of economies of scale. Several of the studies, for example, make the mistake of assuming variable costs are the same per patient at any volume, thus assuming that there are no potential savings from increasing the efficiency of variable inputs via an increase in the volume (Finkler, 1979; Finkler, 1981 and McGregor and Pelletier, 1978). These studies are therefore assigned a zero validity weight.

Munoz et al (1990a,b,c) applied a simple statistical methodology to study the existence of economies of scale in the treatment of urology, orthopaedic and neurosurgical patients; surgeons were classified into low and high-volume categories. Costs per patient, adjusted for case-mix and severity of illness (proxy), were lower for higher-volume surgeons. The crude proxy for severity of illness used means that study findings might be due to low-volume surgeons treating more complex – and hence costly – cases. Moreover, some of the physicians under study were full-time staff members whilst others were private practice part-time employees.

If these findings do indeed reflect real effects it is still not clear what they reveal about economies of scale and the optimal configuration of hospital services. If such economies exist they might, for example, be due to a surgical learning curve (see Chapter 2) Other important sources of economies or diseconomies of scale that might arise through an increased concentration of services within few large hospitals are ignored. For example, economies due to indivisibilities in medical equipment or uncertain demand are not measured in such study designs. Nor are the diseconomies related to management that could arise in larger hospitals.

A study that could deserve more attention is the flexible cost model by Okunade (1993) exploring the cost structure of hospital pharmacies. In the one-output, multiple-input translog model, slight but statistically significant short-run diseconomies of scale are found at the sample means. The most efficient operating size in the short-run is the median bed size category of 200–299 beds.

This study and all the other studies mentioned in this section share a common limitation; they assume that hospital production is separable, that is, that hospitals do not use their inputs to produce joint products (e.g. one piece of medical equipment to be used for two different specialities). Yet it might be expected that

the cost of providing – for instance – maternity care might increase if a hospital eliminates its main paediatric service.

3.8 EVIDENCE FROM MULTI-HOSPITAL ARRANGEMENTS

A separate literature has been concerned with the impact of various forms of consolidation on hospital performance. A central question is whether the motive for the observed mergers or other multi-hospital arrangements in the US was increased operating efficiencies or instead more aggressive pricing policies and the exploitation of monopoly power. Operating efficiency was primarily examined in terms of changes in cost per case or per day and in productivity indices following a new arrangement. With the exception of the study by Sinay (1994), this literature at best fails to identify the portion of the change in average cost that is attributable to economies of scale as opposed to scope effects, and *vice versa*. At worst, other uncontrolled factors (e.g. a change in pure technical efficiency) due to the radical restructuring of hospitals following the merger or changes in accounting practice might be partly or wholly responsible for any change in cost per case (Sinay, 1997; Mobley, 1990). Or it could be, as Manheim, et al (1989) note, that efficiencies are gained by improving the management of a hospital acquired by an investor-owned chain. Although a detailed review of the mergers literature falls beyond the scope of this study, it is still useful to examine some of the findings.

Empirical studies have used basically two methodologies to examine the important issue of hospital performance. The first is the statistical technique, which constructs pairs of matched independent and system-affiliated (or merged) hospitals for relevant factors other than the ones of interest. Performance indicators, such as adjusted average cost per case, can then be compared across the matched samples. Levitz and Brook (1985) found that cost per case adjusted for case-mix intensity was significantly higher for system-affiliated hospitals. Treat (1976) found that the average cost per case after mergers was higher for urban but lower for rural hospitals, suggesting that efficiency can only be improved through mergers of small rural units. However, the findings cannot be solely attributed to the presence of economies or diseconomies of scale (or better to a combination of scope and scale effects). Pattison and Katz (1983) also found investor-owned chain hospitals to have a higher cost per case than free-standing voluntary institutions, attributing the enhanced profitability of the former to the aggressive marketing and pricing strategies used rather than to cost savings. Similar results, though based on cost per day, were obtained by Lewin et al (1981).

This methodology has been criticised for its inability to control for the effects of many potential confounding factors affecting hospital performance. Multiple regression has thus been suggested as a more appropriate design. Average cost per case is regressed on control variables and a dummy variable indicating hospital type from a sample of hospitals including independent hospitals as well as members of multi-hospital systems.

Coyne (1982) runs separate cost per case regressions for different hospital ownership types (religious, other non-profit, investor-owned, county) and controls for differences in case-mix, demography, competition and regulation. System hospitals of all ownership types are shown to incur higher unit costs except for county-owned system hospitals, which instead have lower cost per case (R^2 0.79–0.98). Becker and Sloan (1985) also found no conclusive evidence that system hospitals are more efficient than independents, after controlling for case-mix and other factors. Mobley (1990) suggested that past research suffered inadequate adjustment for a number of factors affecting average cost (e.g. case-mix, quality, increased insurance market competition). This model, however, did not find any significant evidence that economies of multi-plant operation (economies of scope included) existed for system hospitals.

The failure of multi-hospital arrangements to achieve lower unit costs is also supported by the reviews of Ermann and Gabel (1986) and Markham (1995). Thus, the merger literature might suggest that in practice economies of scale and scope at the hospital level are not realised in such arrangements. The evidence however is also in line with our earlier results that economies are probably absent for medium and large-sized hospitals.

Sinay (1994) tested the hypothesis that hospital mergers in the 1980s reduced production costs by achieving economies of scale and scope by comparing merged hospitals with a control group of non-merged hospitals matched for location, ownership and system status, size, and services provided. The author claims to have found that merged hospitals eventually managed to exploit economies in one merger episode. However, the results do not seem to be conclusive about the optimum: in the other episode studied, merged hospitals experienced diseconomies prior to the merger but (unexploited) economies two years after when the average hospital size in the sample increased from 229 to 429 beds. Moreover, the model employs the day as the unit of output and adjusts crudely for input prices.

Finally, it is worth noting that there might be alternative motives for multi-hospital arrangements, such as reputation benefits (Dranove and Shanley, 1995).

3.9 CONCLUSIONS AND IMPLICATIONS FOR THE NHS

Economies of scale for general hospitals have been examined extensively by econometric flexible cost models. The more reliable studies find constant returns or even diseconomies for the average hospital: one with roughly 200–300 beds. If any economies exist they appear to be quickly exhausted or outweighed by diseconomies. Hospitals of 400 beds or more might be too large with respect to cost minimisation or at best no more beneficial than smaller units. The absence of cost savings from expanding the scale of production is corroborated by ad hoc cost models. These are in general less reliable than flexible cost functions but have used a larger number of case-mix variables. The production function approach confirms these findings.

Data Envelopment Analysis (DEA) reinforces the view that economies can be exploited only up to a hospital size of about 200 beds. It also suggests that hospitals larger than some 650 beds are scale-inefficient. Results are conflicting regarding the exact position of the optimum, but it may lie between 200 and 400 beds. It is encouraging that these findings are not very different from those in flexible econometric models, since both techniques have different relative strengths and weaknesses.

Survival analyses are less reliable mainly because it is more difficult to identify and control for factors, other than size, that affect survival, as indicated by the low R^2 found in such studies. Yet they have been seen as a complementary tool in the analysis of economies, in light of the potential biases that arise from analyses using hospital data. Unexploited economies are again reported for hospitals with fewer than 200 beds. It is less clear however, whether diseconomies ever set in and whether hospitals within the 200–300 range can still exploit further cost savings. The findings of the literature focusing on the hospital level are also broadly in line with the evidence provided by studies examining the impact of mergers and other multi-hospital arrangements on costs.

Econometric hospital cost studies have also been used to examine the existence of economies of scope. Their existence was not in general empirically validated for the average hospital, but this does not necessarily mean that they are absent. Some questionable evidence exists that there might be some economies between obstetrics and medical (acute) care and between acute and sub-acute care.

Reliable estimates of economies can only be obtained, in principle, if all other relevant factors are adequately controlled for, which is extremely difficult. Other limitations of the existing literature have also been identified. Thus, all evidence reported in this chapter should be interpreted with a degree of caution.

What are the implications of the available evidence for the NHS? The specific issue of interest here is whether increasing concentration by, for example, hospital mergers can be expected to generate cost savings in the NHS through the exploitation of economies of scale. The literature which deals directly with this question (mostly from the USA) is inconclusive, but there is no support for the presumption that unit costs are lower in multi-hospital systems, or that a merger automatically reduces costs. If, as the research evidence suggests, economies of scale are exhausted at relatively low levels, mergers cannot be expected to offer opportunities for improvements in efficiency when the constituent hospitals are already above the threshold level. The same principle applies to the rationalisation of specialities to a single site.

This is a conclusion which may appear counter-intuitive. Trust mergers, for example, are expected at least to eliminate duplication and to reduce the costs of administration and management. But this, if it happens at all, may be a partial effect. The relevant measure is the change in total costs per episode and not (for example) the change in management costs alone. Assuming the hospital is otherwise efficient, the evidence from the literature predicts that as scale is increased, even though management costs may be reduced, total costs will remain constant or will increase. This could be due to a decline in standards of management leading to reduced efficiency, to a redistribution of management tasks to non-traditional managers, so reducing output, or to the use of more expensive technology.

It is important, however, to recognise that most of the literature on economies of scale is directly relevant only to those hospitals which are technically efficient: that is, are operating on the 'efficiency frontier'. All this evidence can tell us is whether a hospital with 250 beds (which was efficiently operated) would have higher or lower unit costs if it expanded to 400 beds and was equally efficient. Evidence of insignificant opportunities for reducing costs through economies of scale is not in itself a conclusive argument against concentration. Where there is excess capacity, concentration (or merger) may (but need not) reduce overall unit costs by reducing surplus capacity. Altern- atively, where existing facilities are in need of modernisation or refurbishment, a capital scheme involving the concentration or merger of more than one site may offer the most efficient or feasible solution. In those cases it is not the increase in size or concentration that results in an increase in efficiency but, for example, the reduction of excess capacity.

3.10 APPENDIX: CRITERIA USED TO ASSESS STUDY VALIDITY

3.10.1 Ad hoc studies

The validity of each study is assessed according to a set of criteria:

1. **The unit of measurement of hospital output:** the cost per case is superior to the cost per day. The anomalous behaviour of cost per day in conjunction with the higher adjusted R^2 found in the cost-per-case models suggests that the case should be used as the unit of measurement of output.
2. **Choice of functional form:** the Cobb–Douglas form has been found to outperform the quadratic on empirical grounds. However, it makes more restrictive assumptions and hence is less reliable than the flexible functional forms.
3. **Adjustment for heterogeneity of output:** if case-mix is not adequately controlled for, then a finding of diseconomies could be due to the fact that larger hospitals tend to admit more severe (and hence costly) cases. Similar arguments hold for observed scope effects. Adjusting for differences in cases treated seems preferable to adjusting for differences in the services used, since the latter are inputs for the former. The case-mix-adjusted cost equations have empirically higher explanatory power. The more disaggregated the output categories used, the more reliable may be the results.
4. **Derivation of long-run scale estimates:** have studies explicitly followed the formal procedure defined by economic theory for deriving true long-run economies of scale?
5. **Inclusion of input prices:** microeconomic theory states that cost is a function of outputs and input prices. If these are omitted or included in an aggregated way, then the scale and scope estimates might be biased.
6. **Treatment of uncertainty:** larger hospitals are required to hold a smaller proportion of their beds on reserve in order to be able to meet an unanticipated demand for their services. An equal proportionate increase in hospital size and average daily census brings about a rise in this reserve margin (reservation quality).
7. **Adjustment for quality of care:** studies should correct for differences in the quality of care if a similar problem to the case-mix issue is to be avoided.
8. **Choice of model variables:** since the hospital is a complex organisation, there is no single theoretical model explaining its behaviour. This means that it is not clear which variable should enter the cost function. Thus, empirical evidence from hospital cost functions should be viewed with a degree of scepticism.

3.10.2 Flexible cost studies

Five of the criteria that are used to evaluate the validity of the empirical evidence from flexible cost functions are the same as those used for ad hoc functions discussed above (criteria 1, 3, 4, 5 and 6).

Two others are:

9. **Regulatory environment and cost minimisation:** studies that utilise samples of hospitals financed prospectively might be more reliable than those using data from retrospective reimbursement regimes, simply because the cost-minimisation hypothesis assumed by cost functions is more likely to hold.
10. **Regular behaviour of the estimated cost functions:** the reliability of estimates of scale or scope effects depends on whether the estimated cost equations satisfy the so-called regularity condition, such as positive fitted marginal costs for all outputs.

3.10.3 Data envelopment analysis

An additional criterion is:

11. **Sensitivity analysis:** several suggestions have been made in the literature in order to remedy the problems of poor specification

and measurement error which may have very serious effects on the estimates of scale efficiency including *inter alia* stochastic DEA (Banker (1989), or sensitivity analysis (Nunamaker (1985), Valdmanis (1992), and Grosskopf and Valdmanis (1987)). The latter solution entails subjecting the model to different sets of variables and specifications to check whether findings are robust or dependent on the variables chosen.

REFERENCES

Banker R D 1984 Measuring Most Productive Scale Size Using Data Envelopment Analysis. European Journal of Operational Research, 17:35–44.

Banker R D, Conrad, R F, Strauss, R P 1986 A Comparative Application of Data Envelopment Analysis and Translog Methods: An Illustrative Study of Hospital Production. Management Science, 32, no 1, 30–44.

Banker R D 1989 Econometric Estimation and Data Envelopment Analysis. Research in Governmental and Nonprofit Accounting, 5:231–243.

Banks D A 1993 Voluntary and Proprietary Hospital Behavioural Response to Socio-Economic Stimuli. Applied Economics, 25:853–868.

Bays C W 1980 Specification Error in the Estimation of Hospital Cost Functions. Review of Economics and Statistics, 62, no 2, 302–305.

Bays C W 1986 The Determinants of Hospital Size: A Survivor Analysis. Applied Economics, 18:359–377.

Becker E R, Sloan, F A 1985 Hospital Ownership and Performance. Inquiry (USA), 23, no 1, 21–36.

Brown M C 1980 Production and Cost Relations of Newfoundland's Cottage Hospitals. Inquiry (USA), 17:268–277.

Burns A M 1982 The Economics of the Connecticut Hospital Industry: Competition, Structure, and Performance. Unpublished PhD Dissertation, The University of Connecticut.

Butler J R G 1995 Hospital Cost Analysis. Kluwer Academic Publishers, Dordrecht / Boston / London.

Byrnes P, Valdmanis V 1994 Analyzing Technical and Allocative Efficiency of Hospitals. In A Charnes, W W Cooper, A Y Lewin and L M Seiford (eds) Data Envelopment Analysis: Theory, Methodology and Applications Kluwer.

Coyne J S 1982 Hospital Performance in Multihospital Systems: A Comparative Study of System and Independent Hospitals. Health Services Research, 17, no 4 (Winter), 303–329.

Derveaux B, Leleu H, Lebrun T, Boussemart J P 1994 Construction d' un Indice de Productivite pour le Secteur Hospitalier Public, Version Provisoire, Xvemes Journees des Economistes de la Sante, 20 et 21 Janvier.

Dranove D, Shanley, M 1995 Cost Reductions or Reputation Enhancement as Motives for Mergers: The Logic of Multihospital Systems. Strategic Management Journal, 16:55–74.

Eakin K B, Kniesner T J 1988 Estimating a Non-minimum Cost Function for Hospitals. Southern Economic Journal, 54:583–597.

Ermann D, Gabel J 1986 Multihospital Systems: Issues and Empirical Findings, Health Affairs. 3, no 1 (Spring), 50–64.

Evans R G, Walker H D 1972 Information Theory and the Analysis of Hospital Cost Structure. Canadian Journal of Economics, 5, no 3, 398–418.

Feldstein M S 1967 Economic Analysis for Health Ser-vices Efficiency: Econometric Studies of the British National Health Service. North-Holland Publ Co, Amsterdam.

Feldstein M S, Schuttinga J 1977 Hospital Costs in Massachusetts: A Methodological Study, Inquiry (USA). 14 (March), 22–31.

Finkler S A 1979 Cost–Effectiveness of Regionalization: The Heart Surgery Example. Inquiry, 16 (Fall), 264–270.

Finkler S A 1981 Cost–Effectiveness of Regionalization: Further Results for Heart Surgery. Health Services Research, 16, no 3 (Fall), 325–333.

Frech H E III, Mobley L R 1995 Resolving the Impasse on Hospital Scale Economies: A New Approach. Allied Economics, 27:286–296.

Gaynor M, Anderson G F 1995 Uncertain Demand, the Structure of Hospital Costs, and the Cost of Empty Hospital Beds. Journal of Health Economics, 14: 291–317.

Grosskopf S, Valdmanis V 1987 Measuring Hospital Performance: A Non-parametric Approach. Journal of Health Economics, 6:89–107.

Gruca T S, Nath, D 1994 Regulatory Change, Constraints on Adaptation and Organisational Failure: An Empirical Analysis of Acute Care Hospitals. Strategic Management Journal, 15:345–363.

Jensen G A, Morrisey M A 1986 The Role of Physician in Hospital Production. Review of Economics and Statistics, 63, no 3, 432–442.

Kemere P 1992 The Structure of Hospital Costs: An Econometric Analysis of Short-term General Hospitals in Maryland. Unpublished PhD Dissertation, Howard University, Washington, DC.

Lavers R J, Whynes D K 1978 A Production Function of English Maternity Hospitals. Socio-economic Planning Sciences, 12, no 2, 85–93.

Levitz G S, Brooke P P Jr 1985 Independent versus System-Affiliated Hospitals: A Comparative Analysis of Financial Performance, Cost and Productivity. Health Services Research, 20, no 3, 315–339.

Lewin L S, Derzon R A, Margulies, R 1981 Investor-owners and Nonprofits Differ in Economic Performance. Hospitals (July), 52–58.

Lillie–Blanton M, Felt S, Redmon P, Renn S, Machlin S, Wennar, E 1992 Rural and Urban Hospital Closures, 1985-1988: Operating and Environmental Characteristics that Affect Risk. Inquiry, 29 (Fall), 332–344.

Lynch J R, Ozcan Y A 1994 Hospital Closure: An Efficient Analysis. Hospital and Health Services Administration, 39, no 2, 205–220.

Maindiratta A 1990 Largest Size-Efficient Scale and Size Efficiencies of Decision-Making Units in Data Envelopment Analysis. Journal of Econometrics, 46:57–72.

Manheim L M, Shortell, S M McFall, S 1989 The Effect of Investor-Owned Chain Acquisitions on Hospital Expenses and Staffing. Health Services Research, 24, no 4, 461–484.

Markham B 1995 Review of the Multi-hospital Arrangements Literature: Benefits, Disadvantages, and Lessons for Implementation. Submitted to Forum.

McGregor M, Pelletier G 1978 Planning of Specialized Health Facilities: Size vs Cost and Effectiveness in Heart Surgery. The New England Journal of Medicine, 299: 179.

Mobley L R, 1990 Multihospital Systems in California: Behaviour and Efficiency. Unpublished PhD Dissertation, University of California, Santa Barbara.

Mobley L R, Frech H E III 1994 Firm Growth and Failure in Increasingly Competitive Markets: Theory and Application to Hospital Markets. Journal of the Economics of Business, 1, no 1, 77–93.

Montfort G van 1981 Production Functions for General Hospitals. Social Science and Medicine, 15C: 87–98.

Mulligan J G 1987 Hospital Scale Economies due to Stochastic Demand and Service. Economic Letters, 23, no 2, 193–197.

Munoz E, Boiardo R, Mulloy K, Goldstein J, Brewster J G, Tenenbaum N, Wise L 1990a Economies of Scale, Physician Volume for Orthopedic Surgical Patients, and the DRG Prospective Payment System. Orthopaedics, 13, no 1 (Jan), 39–44.

Munoz E, Boiardo R, Mulloy K, Goldstein J, Tenenbaum N, Wise L 1990b Economies of Scale, Physician Volume for Neurosurgery Patients, and the Diagnosis-Related Group Prospective Hospital Payment System. Neurosurgery, 26, no 1 (Jan), 156–161.

Munoz E, Boiardo R, Mulloy K, Goldstein J, Brewster J G, Wise, L 1990c Economies of Scale, Physician Volume for Urology Patients, and DRG Prospective Hospital Payment System. Urology, XXXVI, no 5 (Nov), 471–476.

NHS Centre for Reviews and Dissemination 1996 Undertaking Systematic Reviews of Research on Effectiveness: CRD Guidelines for Those Carrying Out or Commissioning Reviews. CRD Report Number 4. University of York.

NHS Centre for Reviews and Dissemination 1997 The relationship between volume and the scope of activity and hospital costs. CRD Report Number 8 part III. University of York.

Nunamaker T R 1985 Using Data Envelopment Analysis to Measure the Efficiency of Non-profit Organizations: A Critical Evaluation. Managerial and Decision Economics, 6, no 1, 50–58.

Okunade A A 1993 Production Cost Structure of USA Hospital Pharmacies: Time-Series, Cross-sectional Bed Size Evidence. Journal of Applied Econometrics, 8: 277–294.

Pangilinan M-B 1991 Production / Cost Inefficiency and Flexible Cost Functions: The Case of New York State Hospitals, 1981-1987. Unpublished PhD Dissertation, State University of New York at Albany.

Pattison R V, Katz H M 1983 Investor-Owned and Not-For-Profit Hospitals: A Comparison Based on California Data. The New England Journal of Medicine, 309, no 6, 347–353.

Pauly M V 1978 Medical Staff Characteristics and Hospital Costs. Journal of Human Resources, supplement, 77–111.

Rozek R P 1988 A Nonparametric Test for Economies of Scope. Applied Economics, 20: 653–663.

Scuffham P A, Devlin N J, Jaforullah M 1996 The Structure of Costs and Production in New Zealand Public Hospitals: An Application of the Transcendental Logarithmic Variable Cost Function. Applied Economics, 28: 75–85.

Simpson J 1995 A Note on Entry by Small Hospitals. Journal of Health Economics, 14: 107–113.

Sinay U A 1994 The Theory of Hospital Mergers: Multiproduct Scope and Scale Economies. Unpublished PhD Dissertation, Saint Louis University.

Sinay U A 1997 Efficiency considerations of hospital mergers: savings in capital and labor costs. Presented at the Association of Health Services Research, Chicago.

Treat T F 1976 The Performance of Merging Hospitals. Medical Care, XIV, no 3, 199–209.

Valdmanis V 1992 Sensitivity Analysis for DEA Models: An Empirical Example using Public vs NFP Hospitals. Journal of Public Economics, 48: 185–205.

Vita M G 1990 Exploring Hospital Production Relationships with Flexible Functional Forms. Journal of Health Economics, 9: 1–21.

Vita M G, Langenfeld J, Pautler P, Miller L 1991 Economic Analysis in health-care Antitrust. Journal of Contemporary Health, Law and Policy, 7: 73–115.

4

Access and the utilisation of healthcare services

Roy Carr-Hill, Michael Place, John Posnett

4.1 INTRODUCTION

The focus of this chapter is on the relationship between patient access and the utilisation of healthcare services. The national context is one in which health authorities and trusts are facing increasing pressure to concentrate services in order to achieve the (presumed) benefits of economies of scale, and in which reports such as the report of the Expert Advisory Group on Cancer (otherwise known as the 'Calman Report') have recommended the concentration of clinical expertise into specialist cancer centres and units. As services become more concentrated, the effects of reduced access on utilisation and health outcomes is of potential concern.

The evidence which is reported here draws heavily on a systematic review of literature covering the period 1970–1996 (Place, 1997) and on work by Carr-Hill and others on rurality and on the socio-economic determinants of healthcare utilisation. Most of the literature in this area concentrates on the relationship between observed rates of utilisation and *distance* or *travel time* as a proxy for access. Most of the published studies are cross-sectional studies, many of which are poorly adjusted for the effects of confounding. For this reason the evidence needs to be viewed with a degree of caution.

4.2 ACCESS AND THE DETERMINANTS OF UTILISATION

From the point of view of the individual a decision to use healthcare services will be a function of three variables: (i) the opportunity costs of utilisation; (ii) the perceived severity of the condition (relative to 'normal' health) and

(iii) the expected effectiveness of treatment. Other things being equal, the greater the costs of access, the less severe the condition and the less effective the treatment, the lower will be the observed rate of utilisation.

In the context of the NHS *access* is primarily about the social and economic costs of use. Social costs include those costs associated with inconvenient opening hours (e.g. for those in work) or particular costs imposed on users from different ethnic backgrounds (such as language barriers). Economic costs include user charges, travel costs and the opportunity costs of time spent in travelling or in waiting to be seen. The greater the costs of utilisation, the less accessible the service.

With few exceptions secondary healthcare in the NHS can only be accessed by referral from primary care (accident and emergency referral is an exception). Any investigation of the relationship between access and utilisation should start at this point. There are (at least) two important issues here: (i) restricted access to primary care will, *ceteris paribus*, reduce access to secondary care; and (ii) to the extent that general practitioners are influenced in their referral behaviour by the accessibility of services to their patients (the agency relationship might imply that they should be), rates of *referral* to secondary care may be expected to be lower where access costs are high.

The distinction between referral and utilisation is important. The relative accessibility of healthcare services is expected to have an impact at three levels: (i) on the initial decision by the patient to consult (to seek primary diagnosis); (ii) on the decision by the general practitioner to refer for secondary care (or the consultant in the case of referral for tertiary care); and (iii) on the patient's decision to comply with treatment.

Given the proposed determinants of utilisation, increasing the costs of access is likely to have its greatest impact on the initial decision to consult, or on the use of diagnostic services (including primary-care consultation, screening and some out-patient services) more generally. This is because patients are more likely to perceive the benefits of care after diagnosis than in the symptomatic or pre-symptomatic stages of disease. In this context, access to primary care is one of the most important dimensions of accessibility in the NHS.

High costs of access to secondary or tertiary-care services are expected to have a lower impact in deterring referral and compliance because, assuming treatment is perceived to be effective, the expected benefits of healthcare are more likely to offset these costs. However, it is important to recognise that when the costs of access are increased the effect is to shift some of the costs of healthcare from the NHS to patients and their carers. The response to this increase in cost is not expected to be uniform across different sections of the population, and studies which detect no aggregate effect on utilisation may mask significant differences within particular groups, such as those with low personal mobility (Bentham et al, 1985) or those in particular socio-economic groups.

4.3 THE DECISION TO CONSULT

In the NHS, patients have direct access to healthcare services in two ways: by presentation at an Accident and Emergency department (A&E) and by consulting their general practitioner. Evidence suggests that in both cases the decision to consult is affected by accessibility (as measured by distance). In particular, rates of utilisation are expected to be lower for those living further from the service. Since access to secondary-care services in the NHS is through referral from primary care, reduced rates of consultation may lead to delays in referral and to more severe symptoms on presentation, both of which may affect outcomes in serious cases.

4.3.1 Primary care

In Australia, a survey reported by Veitch (1995) indicated that illness behaviour is affected by the perceived severity of the illness and the distance (extending to more than 100 kilometres) from medical care. Willingness to seek care declined with distance, but less so as the severity of the condition increased. Parkin (1979) found that consultation rates in Lambeth declined significantly for patients living more than 5/8 of a mile from their GP. In North West Norfolk, Bentham et al (1992) found that the introduction of a mobile branch surgery into a village nine miles from the main surgery significantly increased the number of patients consulting their doctor.

At an inner-city health centre in Salford, Whitehouse (1985) found that patients from more than two miles away consulted less often, and in the case of women were less likely to have seen their doctor at all. Jones (1996) found that for England and Wales increased mortality was associated with less accessible GPs in the case of malignant neoplasm of the female breast (but not in the case of malignant neoplasm of the cervix uteri). Simon et al (1973) found that fewer students used the student health-service clinic at the University of Rochester after it had been moved to a more distant (over half a mile away) and less accessible location.

In France, Launoy et al (1992) found more severe symptoms on presentation among the rural population (especially women), and this may be indicative of the fact that in some circumstances the effect of reduced access is to delay consultation until symptoms become more severe.

It has long been accepted in the NHS that rurality (and/or distance) will affect the use of general practice services, and this is the rationale for the rural practice allowance which is designed to compensate, in some part, for the additional access costs facing patients by increasing the funding for GPs working in rural areas. However, it remains an open question whether rurality represents an additional barrier to use, independently of distance. The *a*

priori expectation is that it will, primarily because poorer (slower) roads and a lack of public transport in rural areas are expected to make the (time) costs of access associated with a given distance higher.

Data from the Fourth National Morbidity Study of General Practices (MSGP4) can be used to examine the association between both the distance of the patient from a practice and rurality (Royal College of General Practitioners et al 1995). Some illustrative results are shown in Tables 4.1–4.4.

A breakdown of consultation rates in general practice by distance from the surgery (Table 4.1) shows that there is, in general, a gradient with distance, with the main effect being between those living less than 2 km and more than 2 km from the practice. However, for all age groups those living in rural Enumeration Districts (EDs) consult less than those living in urban areas and this is true (with one exception) for consultations for serious reasons and consultations for minor reasons (Table 4.2). These results show evidence of reduced rates of primary-care consultation as distance from the practice increases, and for those living in rural areas.

It is not possible on the basis of this evidence alone to establish whether rurality exerts an independent influence on utilisation. However, a more detailed breakdown suggests that there is no independent effect once distance has been taken into account. Table 4.3 shows consultation rates by age and distance for rural EDs only. The same shallow gradient with

Table 4.1 Consulation rates by age group and distance for . . .

	Distance km	Any reasons M	F	Serious reasons M	F	Minor reasons M	F
Under 5	<2	5.08	4.78	0.35	0.25	2.53	2.40
	2–5	4.56	4.46	0.29	0.24	2.29	2.18
	>5	4.42	4.11	0.28	0.26	2.07	1.89
5–15	<2	2.23	2.53	0.25	0.18	1.00	1.20
	2–5	1.96	2.24	0.20	0.15	0.88	1.04
	>5	1.93	2.33	0.22	0.20	0.83	1.01
16–64	<2	2.51	4.91	0.42	0.49	1.08	2.52
	2–5	2.43	4.42	0.42	0.45	1.04	2.26
	>5	2.18	4.05	0.36	0.41	0.94	2.00
65+	<2	5.23	5.74	1.65	1.51	1.67	1.91
	2–5	4.78	5.10	1.46	1.31	1.48	1.71
	>5	4.71	5.23	1.55	1.46	1.45	1.66

Table 4.2 Consulation rates by age group and distance for . . .

		Any reasons		Serious reasons		Minor reasons	
		M	F	M	F	M	F
Under 5	Urban	4.96	4.69	0.34	0.25	2.47	2.35
	Rural	4.62	4.51	0.27	0.24	2.23	2.09
5–15	Urban	2.17	2.47	0.24	0.17	0.97	1.17
	Rural	2.01	2.34	0.20	0.19	0.86	1.04
16–64	Urban	2.51	4.82	0.42	0.48	1.08	2.47
	Rural	2.21	4.09	0.36	0.41	0.94	2.05
65+	Urban	5.10	5.61	1.61	1.48	1.62	1.86
	Rural	4.99	5.35	1.54	1.39	1.53	1.80

distance, most marked between those living less than 2 km and more than 2 km from the surgery, is evident here as it is in Table 4.1 for the whole population. Although in most cases the rates of consultation are lower than the corresponding rates in Table 4.1 there appears to be no systematic effect for any age or gender group. Consultation rates are actually higher in some cases for those aged under 16. Nonetheless, a separate multivariate analysis on data from the same source suggested that both 'distance from practice in urban areas' and 'residing in a rural Enumeration District' exerted independent effects on rates of consultation (Carr-Hill, Rice and Roland, 1996).

One possible explanation for the fact that rurality appears not to have such a strong effect on utilisation as might be expected is that the percentage of households in rural areas with a car may be higher than in urban areas. Table 4.4 shows a range of Census variables for Enumeration Districts in Herefordshire, for an urban area (Hereford), market towns, villages and 'deep rural' areas (Carr-Hill et al, 1996). There is an evident gradient in some of the conventional indicators of deprivation such as unemployment and lone parents, but the most striking difference is in the percentage of households with no car, which declines from 33 per cent in Hereford to 11.3 per cent in the deep rural areas. Car ownership is one of the ways in which the access costs associated with distance can be reduced.

4.3.2 Accident and emergency

There is evidence of distance-decay in attendances at Accident and Emergency departments. For example, McKee et al (1990) found that in Northern Ireland proximity to an A&E department is associated with increased use. In Bristol, Walsh (1990) found a strong inverse

Table 4.3 Consultation rates by age group and distance: rural EDs only

	Distance km	Any reasons		Serious reasons		Minor reasons	
		M	F	M	F	M	F
Under 5	<2	5.60	5.00	0.45	0.26	2.62	2.35
	2–5	4.32	4.36	0.22	0.20	2.13	2.02
	>5	4.59	4.48	0.27	0.28	2.17	2.06
5–15	<2	2.40	2.45	0.17	0.17	1.02	1.14
	2–5	1.92	2.21	0.21	0.16	0.83	1.00
	>5	1.97	2.50	0.22	0.25	0.82	1.06
16–64	<2	2.02	4.10	0.30	0.37	0.87	2.09
	2–5	2.24	4.07	0.36	0.40	0.96	2.05
	>5	2.28	4.16	0.39	0.44	0.95	2.03
65+	<2	5.16	5.45	1.60	1.44	1.60	1.85
	2–5	5.01	5.23	1.51	1.30	1.54	1.80
	>5	4.86	5.41	1.55	1.52	1.48	1.78

Table 4.4 Proportions of various socio-demographic and 'deprivation' characteristics in electoral EDs in Herefordshire from 1991 Census SAS

	Hereford	Market town	Villages	Deep rural	Herefordshire
No. of EDs	95	59	54	258	466
Over 65+	17.6	22.3	19.3	17.4	18.3
M65 Plus	14.6	18.7	16.5	16.0	16.1
F65 Plus	20.2	25.5	21.7	18.6	20.2
Ethnic	0.9	0.5	0.5	0.3	0.5
Under 5	7.0	6.0	5.9	6.0	6.2
Unemp	8.3	6.6	5.5	5.6	6.3
M unemp	9.8	8.0	6.3	6.0	7.1
F unemp	6.4	4.5	4.3	5.1	5.2
w/o amenities	1.4	0.8	1.1	2.0	1.6
No car	33.0	26.5	14.2	11.3	18.0
Lone parents	4.3	2.2	1.4	1.6	2.2
Elderly alone	15.8	18.2	13.1	12.0	13.7
Not owner occ	36.5	29.7	24.2	28.7	29.9
Unskilled	5.6	5.4	2.5	3.4	4.0

relationship between distance (range 0.7 to 5.8 km) and attendance rates at A&E for those aged 16–60. Bentham et al (1985) found that utilisation of the casualty department in Norwich declined with distance (up to 21 miles) and with reduced personal mobility. In Sweden, Magnusson (1980) observed an inverse relationship between visiting rates to the emergency department and distance (range 5 to 72 minutes travelling time by public transport) which explained 81 per cent of variation in attendance.

In the case of self-referral to A&E departments in West Lothian, Campbell (1994) shows a clear distance-decay effect on referrals (range 0 to 15½ km). However, Campbell found no such association for GP-initiated referral rates. However, in North Worcestershire, Packer et al (1995) found that general medical and geriatric emergency admission rates declined as distance between GP practice and hospital increased.

4.3.3 Screening services

Since screening services are designed to be used by those in the pre-symptomatic stages of disease, it is expected that reduced accessibility will have a negative effect on utilisation. The evidence appears to confirm this hypothesis.

Bentham et al (1995) found that in Norfolk the uptake of opportunistic cervical cytology screening decreased with remoteness. However, remoteness was no longer significant when a new population-based call and recall system was introduced. Haiart et al (1990) found that uptake for a mobile mammography unit operating in East and Midlothian declined with distance from the unit.

In Victoria, Hurley et al (1994) found that the further women had to travel for free mammographic screening the lower the attendance rate. The probability of attending was 0.97^k ($k=1$ kilometre of travel).

The study by Majeed et al (1994) illustrates the fact that distance is not the only important dimension of access. They found that the uptake of cervical smear tests in Merton, Sutton and Wandsworth was greater in larger and computerised practices because they were more likely to have a female GP.

4.4 REFERRAL AND HOSPITAL UTILISATION

4.4.1 Distance and travel time

There are a number of studies which suggest that rates of hospital utilisation are lower in communities living further from hospitals. Our hypothesis leads us to expect that the effect of distance on utilisation will be greatest for those procedures or conditions in which the benefits of treatment are less well established.

In Maine, New Hampshire and Vermont, Goodman et al (1994) found that utilisation of in-patient services for medical DRGs for children under 15 years decays with distance measured as travel time (in the range 0 to 120 minutes). Gittelsohn et al (1995) found that in Maryland distance of more than 80 miles played an important role in determining accessibility for coronary artery bypass graft surgery (CABG) and other discretionary surgery. In France, Launoy et al (1992) found that patients in the Department of Calvados were less likely to receive specialist treatment for colorectal cancer the further they lived from the referral centre.

Wood (1985) found the effects of distance on hospital utilisation in the Grampian region of Scotland to be selective: related both to the distance of the patient from the GP (>3 miles or >5 miles) and the distance of the practice from the hospital (>35 miles). Black et al (1995) examined coronary revascularisations in England and Scotland and found that utilisation increases with the presence of a local cardiologist and decreases with distance from a main specialist centre. Slack et al (1997) found a significant inverse relationship between hospitalisation rates in Bassetlaw and Nottingham and travel times from the patient's ward of residence.

The ratio of the use of in-patient hospital services to need was found to decline with distances of up to 21 miles from Norwich in the study by Bentham et al (1985); they also found that the decline was greatest with reduced personal mobility and with the absence of a local GP surgery.

However, not all of the evidence suggests that distance reduces access. Grumbach et al (1995) compared CABG rates in New York, California, Ontario and British Columbia at distances extending to more than 100 miles: they found that in Canada distance was not associated with lower CABG rates, whereas in the United States the overall rates were higher but were affected by distance-decay. Anderson et al (1989) also found no evidence that rates for CABG in Ontario were affected by distances ranging from 15 to 120 miles. Equally, medical admissions for heart disease in Maryland were not influenced by distance (Gittlesohn et al (1995)). In Manitoba, Roos et al (1985) found that variations in rates of total hip replacement (THR) were not related to distance from the referral centre. They also found no evidence that centralisation had restricted the overall rate of THR.

It is difficult from this evidence alone to identify the separate effects of patient access on the *referral* behaviour of doctors (either general practitioners in the case of secondary services or consultants in the case of tertiary services) and on the willingness of patients to *comply* with medical advice. If doctors act as agents for their patients, then it will be perfectly rational for a doctor's referral decision to be influenced by the same factors which are expected to influence patients themselves. Thus, where the opportunity costs of access are high, doctors may be expected to refer fewer patients than they would if access costs were lower. This deterrence effect is expected to be of less importance where treatment is perceived to be of significant benefit to the patient.

A few studies focus directly on the referral behaviour of doctors: in New Hampshire and Vermont, Greenberg et al (1988) found that referral of lung cancer patients to the University cancer centres was strongly related to the patient's distance from the centres, ranging from less than 25 to more than 75 miles. Roos et al (1989) found an apparent reluctance of physicians in Western Manitoba to refer to Winnipeg for coronary artery bypass graft surgery, even though their own local hospital could not perform the procedures. On the other hand Clarke, et al (1995) found that referrals of patients with testicular cancer to specialist cancer centres were similar throughout Scotland, and that patients living in rural areas had the same chance of referral as other patients.

4.4.2 Access as a supply variable

Although not designed as an investigation of the relationship between access and utilisation, the small area analysis of hospital utilisation carried out in England and Northern Ireland as part of the process of developing a needs-based formula for allocating NHS resources also developed measures of accessibility in order to control for the effects of supply on utilisation (see Carr-Hill et al, 1994, Appendix C for details).

These measures were designed to reflect the accessibility of all beds in England (or Northern Ireland) to the residents of each electoral ward (the analysis is actually based on 'synthetic' wards constructed by combining some of the smaller electoral wards). The aim was to produce a distance-weighted form of the standard beds per thousand ratio, and this weighted measure was computed using spatial interaction modelling assuming an inverse square deterrence function and an intrazonal cost of 10 km (in other words, adding 10 km to all distances before computing the accessibility score).

In the English work (Carr-Hill et al, 1994) four different accessibility measures were created for each ward:

ACCNHS Number of NHS beds weighted by the inverse square of distance (separately for acute and non-acute beds).

ACCGPS Number of general practitioners weighted by the inverse square of distance.

HOMES Proportion of the population not living in nursing or residential homes on Census night.

ACCPRI Number of places in private hospitals on Census night weighted by the inverse square of distance.

For the analysis in Northern Ireland it was possible to compute accessibility measures on the basis of the actual hospital of treatment (O'Reilly et al, 1997):

ACCSURG A distance-weighted ratio of surgical beds per head for each ward, calculated as in the English work.

GERBEDS A distance-weighted ratio of geriatric beds per head for each ward, calculated as in the English work.

SBWRATIO The booked to waiting list ratio of residents of a ward who have had elective surgery.

In this exercise, while it was found that the inverse square deterrence function appeared to

be approximately correct for general medicine, the more specialist services exhibited a flatter relationship with distance (i.e. utilisation was relatively less sensitive to distance). Utilisation rates in cardiac surgery, rehabilitation and nephrology were nearly flat with distance (pp. 33–34).

Both of these analyses were based on a simplified, though conceptually complete, model of the relationship between healthcare utilisation, supply and the relative need for healthcare between local populations (Figure 4.1), and used the technique of two-stage least squares to control for the potentially confounding effect of need on the relationship between utilisation and supply. The results of the work for England can only test the impact of a particular assumed accessibility function (i.e. an inverse square deterrence function with an intrazonal cost of 10 kms), while the work for Northern Ireland allows the function to differ between specialties.

Results for England and Northern Ireland are shown in Tables 4.1A and 4.2A in the Appendix to this chapter. Accessibility is not significant as a determinant of differences in the utilisation of acute beds in either England or Northern Ireland, and this is consistent with the conclusions of most of the literature. However, in England the utilisation of non-acute beds (e.g. psychiatric beds) is significantly associated with access, although the direction of this association is negative: the greater the access, the lower the rate of utilisation. This is a counterintuitive result which is also found in the case of elective surgery in the analysis for Northern Ireland.

It is relevant to note also that access to general practitioners (GPs) is significant in all of the equations shown in Tables 4.1A and 4.2A The relationship is positive, as expected: the greater the access to GPs, the greater the rate of hospital utilisation.

4.5 PATIENT COMPLIANCE

Part of the explanation for lower rates of hospital utilisation in communities living further from health services may be that patients themselves make a decision not to comply with treatment, or with recommended follow-up. If this is a significant determinant of differences

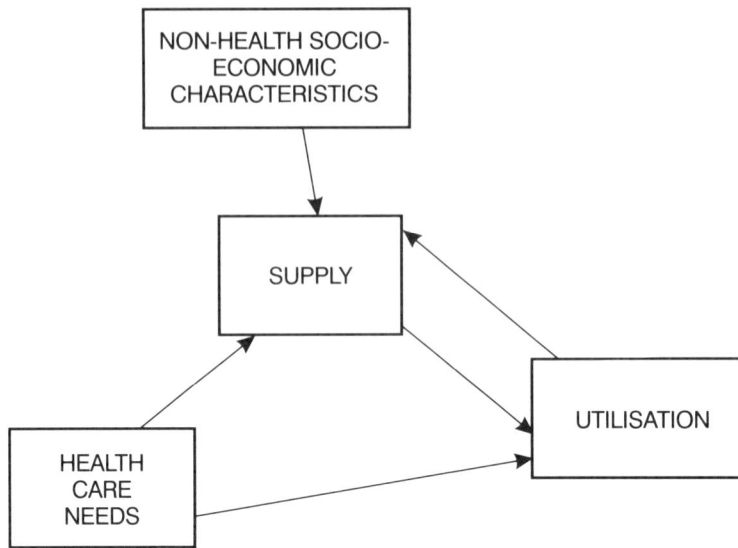

Figure 4.1 A simplified model of demand for healthcare

in rates of utilisation it should be evident in attendance at clinics, at out-patient appointments, or for pre-booked day-case procedures. The evidence is mixed. The deterrent effect of distance appears to vary between services, and in some cases evidence of lower rates of compliance are associated with very large distances (of 100 miles or more) from the service.

Drop-out rates from clinics have been shown to increase with distance in the case of alcoholism after-care in the United States (Fortney et al (1995)). Attendance at after-care sessions for alcoholics in Jackson, Mississippi reduced with distance (range 6–189 miles), and more so for off-highway distance (Prue et al (1979)).

Drop-out rates from clinics have been shown to increase with distances of over 100 miles by Graber et al (1992) for adult diabetics in Nashville. Missed visits in an American ophthalmology clinical trial were found by Orr et al (1992) to be associated with distance (of over 100 miles) and travel costs. Patients more than three miles away were found to miss fewer appointments than those closer to an urban family practice in the American Midwest (Smith et al (1994)).

Haynes et al (1979) found that attendance at out-patient clinics in King's Lynn declined when the distance from home increased to over ten miles. Bentham et al (1985) found that in Norfolk utilisation of out-patients declined with distance (up to 21 miles) from Norwich, and more so for those with reduced personal mobility and those remote from a GP surgery. In Dublin, Kaliszer et al (1981) found that distance from an antenatal clinic affected the timing of the first visit, with those living at a distance of four miles or more presenting three weeks later than those nearby. There was no relationship between distance and missed visits.

On the other hand, Meyers et al (1995) found no correlation between distance, in some cases over 500 km, and non-compliance for paediatric allografts in Johannesburg. Where patients in Lanarkshire required further investigation after initial screening for breast cancer, Kohli et al (1995) found no defaults on appointments: some had considered not attending, but not because of distance, time or cost. Patients were helped by being given convenient appointment times and travel expenses if they were on income support. They had to travel from 14 to 46 miles, taking between 30 minutes and 5½ hours for the return trip. In Glasgow, Junor et al (1992) found no refusals, drop-outs or non-compliance amongst radiotherapy out-patients. Patients perceived the service to be important enough to overcome the barriers of time and distance (range 1 to 60 miles) with the help of hospital and charity transport, or overnight hotel accommodation provided by the hospital where necessary.

Strong et al (1991) audited day case cataract surgery at Leicester Royal Infirmary. They concluded that although 'it might have been expected that geographic factors would affect the decision whether to admit as a day case, our data show this was not the case. Some day case patients travelled over 30 miles each way.'

4.6 ACCESS AND OUTCOMES

To the extent that distance or travel time is a determinant of utilisation, it is natural to look for evidence that health outcomes are actually adversely affected as access is reduced. Unfortunately there is little direct evidence available on the relationship between distance and outcome.

In the case of serious road traffic accidents (RTAs), Jones et al (1995) found that emergency medical service times (of up to 52 minutes from accident to hospital) were not associated with the outcome of RTAs in Norfolk. On the other hand, in Montreal a total pre-hospital time of more than 60 minutes was associated for severely injured patients with a threefold increase in the odds of dying within six days (Sampalis et al (1993)).

In the semi-rural eastern townships of Quebec, Kelly et al (1974) found that households from 10 to over 30 minutes distant from the nearest hospital had significantly more deaths from acute medical post-neonatal syndromes in children under five than did the nearest households, less than 10 minutes away. Jones (1996) found that in England and Wales greater distance (extending to over 22 km) from the nearest hospital was associated with increasing mortality for diabetes mellitus and asthma, and increasing mortality in the first 28 days of life, and in road traffic accidents.

There was no such association for breast cancer, cervical cancer, hypertension and stroke, or peptic ulcer (Jones (1996)); and in Finland, Karjalainen (1990) found that the centralisation of radiotherapy facilities did not appear to have affected the five-year survival rates for patients with breast cancer or prostatic cancer.

4.7 SUMMARY

It is important, in interpreting the findings of published studies, to bear in mind the need to control for factors which may confound an observed association between distance and utilisation. Differences in healthcare needs is an obvious example. A negative empirical relationship between rates of utilisation and distance from provision cannot necessarily be interpreted as evidence of a deterrent effect unless all relevant confounding factors have been controlled. For example, if populations living in inner-city areas close to the site of an acute hospital have higher rates of utilisation than populations from outlying suburbs, this is not conclusive evidence of distance-decay. It may simply be a reflection of the fact that inner-city populations have higher levels of healthcare need.

Bearing in mind these qualifications on the interpretation of published studies, the literature suggests a number of conclusions:

- there is evidence of distance-decay in primary-care consultations for both urban and rural populations, and this is particularly important for health education and for the detection of disease at the symptomatic stage. The evidence from France of more severe symptoms for colorectal cancer at diagnosis amongst the rural population, especially women, may be a result of delayed presentation caused by the costs of access;
- there is also evidence of a negative association between distance and attendance at accident and emergency departments;
- evidence relating to the take-up of screening services indicates a negative effect of distance in the case of both mammography and cervical cytology. Where screening is practice-based, distance from primary care will be relevant;
- There is evidence that distance is associated with reduced rates of attendance at out-patient clinics and at clinics for some specialist services (such as alcoholism after-care), but there is also evidence that attendance for other services, such as radiotherapy or for follow-up investigations following

breast-cancer screening, are not affected by distance in the ranges 14–46 miles (breast screening) and 1–60 miles (radiotherapy);

- there is no evidence of a general relationship between accessibility and the utilisation of acute hospital services, although there is evidence in the literature of a negative association for some specific services (such as CABG and other discretionary surgery, treatment for colorectal cancer and coronary revascularisation). The work on the determinants of utilisation in England and Northern Ireland which suggests a positive effect of distance on the utilisation of non-acute beds and elective surgery is intriguing, if not altogether intuitive;

- some studies identify an independent effect of distance on referrals (e.g. for lung cancer, CABG and cardio-thoracic surgery) which suggests that GPs and other referring physicians may be influenced in their behaviour by the accessibility of services to their patients. On the other hand evidence from Scotland suggest that referrals of patients with testicular cancer to specialist centres are similar in all areas, and one study found that rates of total hip replacement in Manitoba were unrelated to distance from the referral centre. This latter study also suggested that centralisation of services did not adversely affect utilisation.

The distances involved in the limited number of UK studies vary widely. For example, Wood (1985) finds an association between utilisation and distance between GP surgery and hospital (>35 miles) and percentage of practice population within 3 and 5 miles of the surgery. Packer et al. (1995) report a relationship between emergency admission rates and distance between hospital and GP surgery. All but one of the 40 practices in the study were within 8 miles of a hospital. In the study by Bentham et al (1985) the ratio of use of in-patient hospital services to need was found to decline with distance (4–7 miles compared with 15–21 miles from the hospital). Finally, Bagust et al (1991) report higher rates of cardio-thoracic surgery for residents in Newcastle compared with patients from distances of up to 65 miles.

Direct evidence of the relationship between distance and mortality or morbidity is rare. However, a number of studies report a negative relationship between distance and outcomes or health status.

The decision of an individual to use hospital services will be a function of the opportunity cost of access and the perceived benefits of the service. In this context evidence that use of diagnostic services (such as screening, primary-care consultation and some out-patient services) may be more sensitive than treatment services to the costs of access is hardly surprising. Patients are more likely to perceive the benefits of care after diagnosis than in the symptomatic or pre-symptomatic stages of disease. In the case of diagnosed disease, assuming that treatment is perceived as being effective, the potential effect of reduced accessibility on utilisation appears to be small, at least within the range of distances which is reported in the literature.

The moderating effect of general practitioners is important. Restricted access to primary care will, *ceteris paribus*, have a direct effect on referrals to the secondary sector, and there also appears to be evidence that GP referrals (and the referrals of consultants) are influenced by the accessibility of secondary and tertiary services. It is difficult to predict from the existing evidence the extent to which the effects of concentration on utilisation are the result of changes in the referral behaviour of physicians, or changes in the compliance or consultation behaviour of patients.

Finally, where the costs of access are increased the effect is to shift some of the costs of healthcare from the NHS to patients and their carers. The response to this increase in cost is not expected to be uniform across different sections of the population, and studies which detect no overall deterrent effect on utilisation may mask significant effects within particular groups, such as those with low personal mobility (Bentham et al 1985) or those in particular socio-economic groups. The impact of concentration in exacerbating inequality of access to healthcare services is a further important issue which is, as yet, largely unexplored.

4.8 APPENDIX

Table 4.1A Analyses of hospital in-patient utilisation in England

	Acute utilisation			Non-acute utilisation		
	Coefficient	Standard error	T value and significance	Coefficient	Standard error	T value and significance
ACCNHS	0.04	0.048	0.82 (NS)	−0.33	0.128	2.60**
ACCGPS	0.33	0.077	4.32***	0.32	0.081	4.01**
HOMES	0.13	0.062	2.15*	−0.77	0.167	4.58**
ACCPRI	0.11	0.036	3.11**	0.16	0.102	1.56 (NS)

Notes: *   significant at 5% level
        **   significant at 1% level
        ***   significant at 0.1% level

In the model for utilisation of acute services the following variables were also found to be significant:

- density (persons divided by hectares);
- manual (proportion of households with head in manual social classes);
- old alone (proportion of people of pensionable age living alone);
- single carers (proportion of dependants in single carer households);
- unemployment (proportion of economically active unemployed);
- smr0–74 (standardised mortality ratio for ages 0–74).

In the model for utilisation of non-acute services the following variables were also found to be significant:

- lone parent (proportion of households headed by a lone parent);
- no carer (proportion of dependants with no carer);
- minorities (proportion of persons born in New Commonwealth);
- old alone (proportion of people of pensionable age living alone);
- smr0–74 (standardised mortality ratio for ages 0–74);
- permanent sick (proportion of adult population who are permanently sick);
- urbanisation (proportion of population living in 'urban' enumeration districts (as defined by the Department of the Environment);
- students (proportion of 17 year olds who are students).

Table 4.2A Analyses of hospital in-patient utilisation in Northern Ireland

	Acute utilisation				Elective surgery utilisation		
	Coefficient	Standard error	T value and significance		Coefficient	Standard error	T value and significance
ACCNHS	0.02	0.035	0.46	ACCSURG	−0.175	0.084	2.09*
ACCGPS	0.091	0.025	3.59**	GERBEDS	0.058	0.015	3.82***
HOMES	−0.195	0.044	4.40***	SBWRATIO	−0.084	0.048	1.74
ACCPRI	−2.27	1.17	1.94*				

Notes: *   significant at 5% level
        **   significant at 1% level
        ***   significant at 0.1% level

In the model for utilisation of acute services the following variables were also found to be significant:

- over 75s alone (proportion of people over 75 living alone);
- family credit (proportion of households in receipt of family credit);
- income support (proportion of households in receipt of income support);
- low birth weight (proportion of births less than 2,500 gms);
- standardised sickness ratio (permanent sickness standardised for age and sex);
- smr all ages (all ages standardised mortality rate).

In the model for utilisation of elective surgery the following variables were also found to be significant:

- proportion in households not lacking central heating;
- proportion of population not Roman Catholic;
- proportion of those aged 75+ living alone;
- proportion of families not on family credit;
- proportion of over 65s on income support;
- proportion of under 65 working age on income support;
- proportion of households without two cars;
- standardised mortality ratio below 75 years of age;
- Proportion of persons in permanent buildings owner occupied.

REFERENCES

Anderson G M, Lomas J 1989 Regionalization of Coronary Artery Bypass Surgery. Effects on Access. Medical Care. 27:288–96.

Bagust A, Currie E J, Slack R 1991 Options for Developing Cardio-Thoracic Services in the Northern Region. YHEC.

Bentham G, Haynes R 1985. Health, Personal Mobility and the Use of Health Services in Rural Norfolk. Journal of Rural Studies. 1:231–9.

Bentham G, Haynes R 1992 Evaluation of a Mobile Branch Surgery in a Rural Area. Social Science and Medicine. 34:1:97–102.

Bentham G, Hinton J, Haynes R, Lovett A, Bestwick C 1995 Factors Affecting Non-Response to Cervical Cytology Screening in Norfolk, England. Social Science & Medicine. 40:131–5.

Black N, Langham S, Petticrew M 1995 Coronary Revascularisation: Why Do Rates Vary Geographically in the UK? Journal of Epidimiology & Community Health. 49:408–12.

Campbell J L 1994 General Practitioner Appointment Systems, Patient Satisfaction, and Use of Accident and Emergency Services – A Study in One Geographical Area. Family Practice. 11:438–45.

Carr-Hill R A, Hardman G, Martin S, Peacock S, Smith P 1994 A Formula for Distributing NHS Revenues Based on a Small Area Use of Hospital Beds, University of York. Centre for Health Economics.

Carr-Hill R A, Rice N, Roland M 1996 Socio Economic Determinants of Rates of Consultation in General Practice as Fourth National Morbidity Survey of General Practice. BMJ. vol 312, 20 April 1996.

Carr-Hill R A, Sheldon T 1991 Designing a Deprivation Payment for General Practitioners – the UPA(8) Wonderland. BMJ. 302(6773) 393–6.

Carr-Hill R A, Watt I, Ivins C, Brown J 1996 Report to Herefordshire Health Authority: Rural Deprivation, Rural Health and Social Needs in Herefordshire. Centre for Health Economics, University of York, February 1996.

Clarke K, Howard G C W, Elia M H, Hutcheon A W, Kaye S B, Windsor P M, Yosef H M A 1995 Referral Patterns within Scotland to Specialist Oncology Centres for Patients with Testicular Germ Cell Tumours. British Journal of Cancer. 72:1300–2.

Fortney J C, Booth B M, Blow F C, Bunn J Y 1995 The Effects of Travel Barriers and Age on the Utilization of Alcoholism Treatment Aftercare. American Journal of Drug & Alcohol Abuse. 21:391–406.

Gittelsohn A, Powe N R 1995 Small Area Variations in Health Care Delivery in Maryland. Health Service Research. 30:295–317.

Goodman D C, Fisher E S, Gittelsohn A, Chang C H, Fleming C 1994 Why are Children Hospitalized? The Role of Non-Clinical Factors in Pediatric Hospitalizations. Pediatrics. 93:896–902.

Graber A L, Davidson P, Brown A W, McRae J R, Woolridge K 1992 Dropout and Relapse During Diabetes Care. Diabetes Care. 15:1477–83.

Greenberg E R, Dain B, Freeman D, Yates J, Korson R 1988.Referral of Lung Cancer Patients to University Hospital Cancer Centers. A Population-Based Study in Two Rural States. Cancer. 62:1647–52.

Grumbach K, Anderson G M, Luft H S, Roos L L, Brook R 1995 Regionalization of Cardiac Surgery in the United States and Canada: Geographic Access, Choice, and Outcomes. JAMA. 274:1282–9.

Haiart D C, McKenzie L, Henderson J, Pollock W, McQueen D D V, Roberts M M, Forrest A P 1990 Mobile Breast Screening: Factors Affecting Uptake, Efforts to Increase Response and Accessibility. Public Health. 104:239–47.

Haynes R M, Bentham C G 1979 Community Hospitals and Rural Accessibility. Teakfield.

Hurley S F, Huggins R M, Jolley D J, Reading D 1994 Recruitment Activities and Sociodemographic Factors that Predict Attendances at a Mammographic Screening Program. American Journal of Public Health. 84:1655–8.

Jones A P, Bentham G 1995 Emergency Medical Service Accessibility and Outcome from Road Traffic Accidents. Public Health. 109:169–77.

Jones A P 1996 Health Service Accessibility and Health Outcomes. University of East Anglia.

Junor E J, Macbeth F R, Barrett A 1992 An Audit of Travel and Waiting Times for Outpatient Radiotherapy. Clinical Oncology. 4:174–76.

Kaliszer M, Kidd M 1981 Some Factors Affecting Attendance at Ante-Natal Clinics. Social Science and Medicine. 15:421–4.

Karjalainen S 1990 Geographical Variation in Cancer Patient Survival in Finland: Chance, Confounding, or Effect of Treatment? Journal of Epidemiology and Community Health. 44:210–214.

Kelly A, Munan L 1974 Epidemiological Patterns of Childhood Mortality and Their Relation to Distance from Medical Care. Social Science & Medicine. 8:363–7.

Kohli H S, Teo P Y, Howie F M, Dobson H M 1995 How Accessible is the Breast Screening Assessment Centre for Lanarkshire Women? Health Bulletin. 53:153–8.

Launoy G, Le Coutour X, Gignoux, Pottier D, Dugleux G 1992 Influence of Rural Environment on Diagnosis, Treatment, and Prognosis of Colorectal Cancer. Journal of Epidimiology and Community Health. 46:365–367.

Magnusson G 1980 The Role of Proximity in the Use of Hospital Emergency Departments. Sociology of Health and Illness. 2:202–214.

Majeed F A, Cook D G, Anderson H R, Hilton H, Bunn S, Stones C 1994 Using Patient and General Practice Characteristics to Explain Variations in Cervical Smear Uptake Rates. BMJ. 308:1272–6.

McCormick M C, Richardson D K 1995 Access to Neonatal Intensive Care. The Future of Children Low Birth Weight. 5:162–175.

McKee C M, Gleadhill D N, Watson J D 1990 Accident and Emergency Attendance Rates: Variation Among Patients from Different General Practices. British Journal of General Practice. 40:150–3.

Meyers K E, Weiland H, Thomson P D 1995 Paediatric Renal Transplantation Non-Compliance. Pediatric Nephrology. 9:189–92.

O'Reilly D, Carr-Hill R, Jamison J W, Stevenson M R, Reid J, Merriman B, Browne S 1997 Report of a Study to Devise a Formula to Assist in Allocating Resources for Acute Hospital Services Within Northern Ireland. Queens University of Belfast. Health and Health Care Research Unit.

Orr P R, Blackhurst D W, Hawkind B S 1992 Patient and Clinical Factors Predictive of Missed Visits and Inactive Status in a Multicenter Clinical Trial. The Macular Photocoagulation Study Group. Controlled Clinical Trials. 13:40–9.

Packer C 1995 The Waiting List Initiative and Emergency Admissions Working Party. Emergency Admissions to the Alexandra Hospital, Redditch. North Worcestershire Health Authority.

Parkin D 1979 Distance as an Influence on Demand in General Practice. Epidemiology and Community Health. 33:96–9.

Place M 1997 The Relationship Between Concentration, Patient Accessibility and Utilisation of Services. NHS Centre for Reviews & Dissemination, University of York. Report 8 Part III.

Prue D M, Keane T M, Cornell J E, Foy Dw 1979. An Analysis of Distance Variables that Affect Aftercare Attendance. Community Mental Health Journal. 15:149–54.

Roos L L, Sharp S M 1989 Innovation, Centralization, and Growth. Coronary Artery Bypass Graft Surgery in Manitoba. Medical Care. 27:441–52.

Roos N P, Lyttle D 1985 The Centralization of Operations and Access to Treatment: Total Hip Replacement in Manitoba. American Journal of Public Health. 75:130–3.

Royal College of General Practitioners, Office of Population Censuses and Surveys, Department of Health 1995 Morbidity Statistics from General Practice, Fourth National Study 1991–1992. HMSO London. (Series MB5, No 3).

Sampalis J S, Lavoie A, Williams J I, Mulder D S, Kalina M 1993 Impact of On-Site Care, Prehospital Time, and Level of In-Hospital Care on Survival in Severely Injured Patients. Journal of Trauma. 34:252–61.

Simon J L, Barton Smith D 1973 Change in Location of a Student Health Service: A Quasi-Experimental Evaluation of the Effects of Distance on Utilization. Medical Care. 11:59–67.

Slack R, Ferguson B, Ryder S 1997 Analysis of Hospitalisation Rates by Electoral Ward: Relationship to Accessibility and Deprivation Data. Health Services Management Research. 10:24–31.

Smith C M, Yawn B P 1994 Factors Associated with Appointment Keeping in a Family Practice Residency Clinic. Journal of Family Practice. 38:25–9.

Strong N P, Wigmore W, Smithson S, Rhodes S, Woodruff G, Rosenthal A R 1991 Daycase Cataract Surgery. British Journal of Ophthalmology. 75:731–3.

Veitch P C 1995 Anticipated Response to Three Common Injuries by Rural and Remote Area Residents. Social Science and Medicine. 41:5:739–45.

Walsh M 1990 Geographical Factors and A & E Attendance. Nursing Standard. 5:28–31.

Whitehouse C R 1985 Effect of Distance From Surgery on Consultation Rates in an Urban Practice. BMJ. 290:359–62.

Wood P W 1985 Geographical Equity and Inpatient Hospital Care: An Empirical Analysis. Departments of Community Medicine and Political Economy. Health Economics Research Unit. University of Aberdeen.

Note: This chapter is based on fieldwork with the
medical Royal Colleges and specialist societies
which Robin Dowie and David Sykes (Centre for
Health Economics, University of York) carried out
in mid-1996 as part of the study on Concentration
and Choice in the Provision of Hospital Services
commissioned by the Department of Health.

5

Changes in medical training and sub-specialisation: implications for service delivery

Robin Dowie, Hugh Gravelle

5.1 INTRODUCTION

In this chapter we describe the way in which
recommendations of the Royal Colleges and
specialist societies in relation to training and
other issues may have implications for the
structure of the hospital service. We detail the
recommendations, discuss the evidence base
for them and discuss their economic and service rationale. But first, salient features of government policies affecting postgraduate
medical training arrangements and their
impact on hospital trusts are outlined.

5.1.1 Organisation and funding of postgraduate training in NHS hospitals

Medical services in hospital trusts in the United
Kingdom are staffed by two main groups of
doctors: consultants and trainees. Consultants
are usually appointed to tenured career posts
and are clinically autonomous. Trainees receive
time-limited appointments and are clinically
responsible to a consultant supervisor. Non-
consultant career doctors form a third, much
smaller group of hospital doctors.They include
associate specialists, staff doctors, and clinical
assistants.

There are three hospital training grades for
doctors:

- pre-registration house officer (PRHO) grade
  filled by medical graduates completing their
  first year of clinical practice;
- senior house officer (SHO) grade for doctors
  in their second, third or fourth clinical year
  working to complete basic specialist or

general professional training in a clinical specialty;

- specialist registrar (SpR) grade: doctors training as specialist registrars to obtain a 'certificate of completion of specialist training' (CCST). Once awarded a CCST, specialist registrars may be appointed to a consultant post in a hospital trust.

The costs of employing medical trainees in hospital trusts are met from the budget held by postgraduate deans and from the service revenues of the trusts. Postgraduate deans are associated with university medical schools. The postgraduate deans' budgets derive from a national Medical and Dental Education levy (MADEL) imposed centrally on health authority allocations. In England, in 1996/97, MADEL totalled £533 million and almost 98 per cent was allocated to the postgraduate deans under four budget heads: training grades (£400 million), postgraduate centres and study leave (£73 million), deans' departments (£31 million), and public health (£16 million) (NHS Executive 1996).

From the training budget the postgraduate deans in England fund:

- 50 per cent of basic salary costs of all full-time post-registration trainees;
- 100 per cent of basic salary costs for pre-registration trainees;
- all non-recurrent 'costs of training' (e.g. costs associated with appointing staff to hospital training posts);
- 100 per cent of basic salary costs for all part-time (flexible) trainees.

Hospital trusts meet:

- 50 per cent of basic salary costs of all full-time post-registration trainees;
- 100 per cent of 'additional duty hours' (ADHs) paid for both full-time trainees and flexible trainees;
- locum costs associated with sickness, annual leave or vacancy.

In England, the present level of funding via MADEL accounts for less than 50 per cent of the total salary costs of trainees. In Scotland, however, the postgraduate deans fund 100 per cent of basic salaries for all trainees.

5.1.2 Recent Government policies affecting the working arrangements of trainees

Since 1990, a succession of Government policies affecting medical training have been implemented, which will have significant effects on patterns of staffing services in acute hospitals.

1. **The New Deal**. Workload surveys conducted in the mid-1980s showed that doctors in busy specialties, who were on duty for six or seven days during the week, were typically working for 60 to 70 hours (Dowie, 1990). A ministerial working party on junior doctor hours was established in 1990 and new working arrangements for doctors and dentists in training were issued – the 'New Deal' (NHS Management Executive, 1991a). A series of target dates was identified for employing authorities to reduce the maximum average number of contracted hours of duty. Finally, on 1 January 1997, no doctor in training should have been contracted for more than 72 hours of duty weekly, except for specialist registrars whose training would benefit from additional clinical experience, and all doctors in training employed on a full-time basis should not have been expected to work for more than an average of 56 hours a week.

Although in October 1996, three months before the final target date, the NHS Executive considered that a quarter of junior doctors in England had not yet met the requirements of the New Deal, there will be significant consequences for Trusts in the future because they will get fewer hours of service from trainee doctors. To keep medical manpower levels constant they will have to find more junior or senior trainees, thereby increasing the influence of training requirements on service provision, or else increase their numbers of consultants or other career-grade doctors.

2. **Specialist medical training**. In the United Kingdom, hospital medical training, from full registration until completion of higher specialist training, has typically taken from five to ten or eleven years depending upon the specialty. Having completed their training many doctors have then waited for an extended period

before obtaining a consultant position. European Community directives indicate, however, that the minimum training periods for specialties should be three, four, or five years depending upon the specialty.

In 1993, a Government working group, under the chairmanship of the chief medical officer for England, Sir Kenneth Calman, advised the Government on action needed to bring training in the United Kingdom into line with European Community directives. The working group's main recommendations were adopted by the Government and consequently the framework for completing postgraduate training in hospital specialties has been radically altered (Department of Health, 1993).

- There is now a single specialist registrar grade in place of two grades of registrar and senior registrar. (One reason for the extended periods of training in Britain was related to the time doctors spent progressing from one grade to another);
- minimum educational requirements for specialist training, and specialist registrar training programmes for the specialties have been introduced;
- a certificate (CCST) is now awarded to persons satisfactorily completing specialist training in a stated specialty. (Specialist registrars in the medical specialties usually follow a training programme leading to two certificates. Arrangements in other specialties for obtaining dual certification have still to be clarified.)
- the contract for specialist registrars is for six months after the anticipated date for award of CCST, these extra months being referred to as a 'period of grace'. An additional contract is then possible but it will be time-limited. Doctors who have not obtained a consultant post by the time the additional contract finishes must leave the grade. (It is too soon to observe the effects of this regulation.)

The overall effect of these reforms is that doctors will take typically six or seven years from full registration until the award of CCST. But, since it will not be permissible for CCST holders to remain for unlimited periods in the SpR grade, a general reduction in the numbers of senior trainees who are available to perform service activities may be observed. Meantime, the policies for issuing contracts to specialist registrars may cause a 'bottle neck' in the progression of senior house officers to the SpR grade.

3. **Postgraduate deans as negotiators of funding for allocated training numbers**. The Department of Health anticipates that hospital trusts will need to employ greater numbers of consultant staff to compensate for these limitations on the availability of experienced trainees. To ensure a sufficient supply of consultants, the annual intake of new trainees for SpR training will have to be increased. A recently established Specialist Workforce Advisory Committee recommended an allocation of almost 1,600 additional higher specialist trainees for England and Wales above a baseline establishment for hospital specialties for 1996/97 (Executive letter EL(96)18). Moreover, 15 specialties were identified as 'priority specialties' in terms of current recruitment difficulties and they were allocated 1,000 of the 1,600 new training numbers.

Postgraduate deans are expected to achieve full implementation of the targets set for their deaneries in these priority specialties. They received additional funding for the SWAG increase for 1996/97 to supplement the resources available from MADEL, but it was not sufficient to cover all the extra training numbers. So, for all specialties, unused training numbers from 1996/97 are to be carried forward for implementation in 1997/98. In addition, the Specialist Workforce Advisory Committee has recommended a new allocation of 850 training numbers for 1997/98 for which the MADEL budget will fund approximately 250 at 50 per cent per SpR placement (Executive letter EL(97)14). To finance the outstanding numbers, funds are being released by converting trusts' existing training posts for 'senior' senior house officers and visiting registrars into specialist registrar placements. Any conversions have to be agreed with the trusts concerned and cannot be imposed by deans. Individual trusts may be reluctant to comply, however, if they are not compensated by being allocated appropriate placements in SpR training programmes.

4. Policies promoting postgraduate education and medical audit. In 1991 the NHS Management Executive set out 10 principles for the delivery of postgraduate medical education, two of which were explicitly about standards:

- high standards of general and specialist training and of continuing medical education are fundamental to the provision of high quality patient care in the NHS;
- the standards of postgraduate and continuing medical and dental education should be monitored (NHS Management Executive 1991b).

Over the following years many trusts initiated action for raising standards of postgraduate training: doctors in the junior training grades began having educational sessions identified in their timetables (this was already a feature of the timetables of senior house officers who were planning to enter general practice and doctors in higher training programmes); consultants were given additional responsibilities for supervising and counselling trainees; and schemes were developed for consultants to become skilled in performing their educational roles.

Prior to the publication of the 1991 policy statement, the Government had made a substantial commitment to promoting medical audit in hospitals. Over the years from 1989–91 to 1993/94, the Department of Health allocated £161 million in England to support medical audit in the hospital and community health service. A Department of Health review of the English regional programmes in 1992/93 suggested that the great majority of hospital doctors were participating in audit activities (such as developing guidelines, auditing records and reviewing clinical policies, and attending audit training activities) (Stern & Brennan no date).

The rapid expansion of these related activities of medical audit and educational endeavour meant that both trainee and consultant staff in the trusts were diverting increasing amounts of time away from the performance of clinical duties. Some departments in the bigger trusts were able to engage sessional help from doctors working part-time to cover the duties of senior house officers whilst they attended educational or audit meetings. But these arrangements were dependent upon the availability of suitable deputising doctors and financial resources. Whether or not the investment of trusts in directly supporting audit and postgraduate education paid off in terms of improved clinical effectiveness is unknown, since comprehensive evaluations of these policies have not been undertaken.

5. Gender of trainees and flexible training. Women form almost half the establishment of pre-registration house officers, the rate of 49 per cent for 1995 being slightly higher than the 1991 rate of 46 per cent, yet only a third of senior trainees in the specialist registrar grade are women. This suggests that disproportionate numbers of women are either entering general practice or discontinuing, perhaps temporarily, their hospital training for personal or professional reasons.

Efforts have been made in the past few years to foster flexible hospital training for women and men, particularly for senior registrars and career registrars, by introducing national specialty quotas for part-time posts (5 per cent of a specialty's registrar posts) and providing central funding for all new part-time posts for a limited period. However, few trainees were part-time employees in 1995 and the situation had changed very little since 1984. For instance, persons with part-time contracts formed 9.4 per cent of all senior registrars in England in 1984 and 8.5 per cent in 1995 (Department of Health, 1996a and 1996b). This overall rate masked wide inter-specialty variations, with the smallest proportions of part-time trainees being found in surgical specialties.

There is an unmet demand for flexible training. In 1996/97 there were some 313 potential flexible trainees in England who were unable to train flexibly because of resource pressures rather than lack of manpower approval or suitable educational opportunities (NHS Executive, 1996). Funding of basic salary costs and additional duties hours for flexible training posts was fully sourced from MADEL until 1996/97. But, in order to release extra funding in the postgraduate deans' MADEL budget for flexible training, trusts assumed financial responsibility for additional duty hours payments in April 1997.

Even without the new responsibility for additional duty hours payments, trusts generally may not wish to be committed to taking on increasing numbers of flexible trainees. The specialist training programmes for part-time trainees have traditionally taken twice as long to complete as the programmes for their full-time colleagues. (The relevant EC directive states that the total duration and quality of part-time training of specialists are not to be less than those of full-time trainees.) The weekly schedules for flexible trainees have to be carefully organised to ensure a balance of clinical duties and responsibilities. This is probably less easily achieved in smaller hospital units.

5.2 ROYAL COLLEGE RECOMMENDATIONS FOR TRAINING

The responsibility for setting standards for postgraduate training is vested in the universities and General Medical and Dental Councils for pre-registration training, the medical Royal Colleges and their faculties for basic specialist training, and the joint higher training committees of the Royal Colleges for higher specialist training (NHS Management Executive, 1991b). This Section is concerned with post-registration training and the role of the collegiate bodies in maintaining standards.

The Colleges exercise their authority in two ways: by awarding postgraduate qualifications to doctors in training, and by accrediting hospitals for training purposes. The recommendations for training accreditation cover a number of areas:

- contracted hours of duty and hours of work, which should accord with the New Deal;
- exposure to minimum numbers of cases or procedures of particular types;
- opportunities for undertaking outpatient work, ward work, and, where appropriate, work in theatres (operating, anaesthetising);
- levels of adequately trained consultant staff to provide supervision;
- protected study and training time;
- education and training resources, such as library facilities, catering, accommodation and other domestic arrangements.

The criteria most relevant for the number and size of hospitals are those relating to consultants and exposure to a minimum caseload to provide sufficient variety of experience. The minimum size of unit would usually follow from an estimate of typical workload.

5.2.1 Recommendations for senior house officer training

1. **Doctors' clinical experience for postgraduate examinations**. The primary examination for each Royal College's postgraduate qualifications is normally taken whilst the candidate is in the SHO grade. As part of the Calman framework for specialist training, two years became the minimum period for completing basic training in the SHO grade in place of a longer minimum training period. Revised College regulations for basic surgical training stipulate that the two years must include two six-month periods in general surgery with emergency work, and orthopaedics with musculoskeletal trauma. The remaining twelve months are to be spent in approved posts in other acute surgical specialties of the trainees' choice. Under the previous regulations trainces were expected also to obtain experience in accident and emergency (A&E) medicine. During the two years after the introduction of the new regulations, hospital trusts reported that they were having difficulties in recruiting doctors to SHO posts in A&E medicine departments. To get around the problem, some trusts funded unconventional non-training posts for 'trust' doctors.

2. **Trusts' standards of training provided in SHO posts**. The Royal Colleges monitor the standards of training offered in SHO posts through a system of hospital recognition quinquennial visits. The Colleges may grant full approval for a five-year period or limited approval subject to improvements being implemented or they may withdraw training recognition. Doctors who occupy posts from which training recognition has been withdrawn cannot have the clinical experience obtained in those posts recognised for examination purposes. This gives the Colleges considerable influence over trusts, since unrecognised posts

will not be attractive to trainees, part of whose costs are met by the postgraduate deans' budgets rather than by trusts.

A benchmark for assessing the clinical experience of SHO posts in many specialties is the rate of patient throughput, although colleges do not always issue explicit guidance on acceptable minimum levels. Explicit guidance exists, however, for basic surgical training in A&E medicine and general professional training in medicine. A&E medicine departments must have a minimum of 25,000 new attendances per annum dependent on the case-mix, while in adult medicine, no individual senior house officer should normally be responsible for more than 25 in-patients or for fewer than 10.

It is unusual for published criteria to contain references to clinical facilities. With basic surgical training, however, an explicit recommendation was made over the provision of computerised tomography in accident and emergency departments. From January 1996, a CT head scanner must be available 24 hours per day for head injury patients.

5.2.2 Recommendations for specialist registrar training

1. **Curricula for higher specialist training**. During 1995 and 1996, the joint higher training committees, on which are representatives of many specialist societies and associations, prepared curricula for specialist training to meet new regulations on European specialist medical qualifications. The curricula had to be approved by the newly established Specialist Training Authority of the Medical Royal Colleges in terms of content and clinical skills attainment by specialist registrars.

The developers of specialist training curricula had to take into account two important factors: first, there are now statutory minimum training periods for individual specialties (ranging from three years to five years) and secondly, the curriculum for a specialty must cover training in sub-specialty interests. (In certain medical and surgical specialties, the minimum programme length, including flexible periods for sub-specialty training, research or other relevant activity, is six years.)

The task of drawing up outline curricula for sub-specialty training was delegated in many specialties to panels representing sub-specialty interests. In general surgery, for example, eight sub-specialties are recognised, each with a national body, and these bodies provided advice on the general surgery curriculum with respect to the content of sub-specialty training and required parameters of clinical experience.

Opinion differed among curricula developers as to whether or not explicit guidance should be incorporated in the curricula on minimum volumes of procedures for trainees to undertake. The curricula for sub-specialist training in cardiology, and gastroenterology and hepatology, in fact, contain detailed minimum targets of procedures. The curriculum for the specialty of ophthalmology, however, only offers guidance on the amount of clinical exposure trainees should have because the higher specialist training committee for ophthalmology did not wish to commit trainees to any form of apparent contractual undertaking.

Now that the new framework for higher specialist training is settling into place certain weaknesses are being identified. One cause for concern is the limitation on the amount of time available for sub-specialist training after generalist experience is completed. Sub-specialisation in pathology, which is necessary in histopathology and haematology for example, is being threatened by the restrictions placed on the length of training for these disciplines.

2. **Standards of higher specialist training programmes**. To ensure that specialist registrars obtain comprehensive training in both district general hospitals and teaching hospitals, specialist training programmes covering both types of hospital placement are being established. There were previously registrar and senior registrar programmes, but the distinctive feature of the new programmes is that the number of identified training slots in each programme will probably exceed the number of specialist registrars entering the programme. This is to allow specialist registrars flexibility when choosing their sub-specialty interest during the early phase of their higher specialist training.

Consultant teams, which previously depended on a senior trainee to assist with service commitments, will not be able to rely on this help being available regularly in future. Personal training programmes for specialist registrars will be more structured than in the past, with time being protected for educational activities in their weekly timetables. This will also reduce their availability for undertaking clinical duties. To compensate for the loss of help from experienced trainees, trusts may seek either to change the working patterns of existing consultants or to expand the consultant establishment. In terms of throughput in smaller units, this could result in high (and costly) ratios of consultants to patients.

The joint higher training committees are using a visitation system to monitor standards in higher specialist training programmes which is similar to the old system for monitoring senior registrar posts. However, the criteria for assessment may be more explicit. Early versions of the visitation documents suggested that workload volumes are a key determinant. Hospitals with insufficiently large caseloads for generalist or sub-specialty training will be at risk of losing their training recognition unless the services are reorganised.

5.3 ROYAL COLLEGE AND SPECIALIST SOCIETY RECOMMENDATIONS FOR SERVICE PROVISION

For many years the Royal Colleges and specialist societies have issued documents containing recommendations on patterns of service provision within the NHS. The recommendations usually cover target catchment populations, medical staffing patterns for career and training grades, workload targets (but not case-mix targets), inter-professional linkages and staffing levels, and equipment and facilities for treating patients. These recommendations carry less force than those arising from training considerations since they are not backed by the ability to derecognise trusts and thus deprive them of a source of labour.

Tables 5.1 and 5.2 summarise recommenda-

tions on patterns of consultant staffing in district hospitals and regional or sub-regional centres that have been made by Royal Colleges and specialist societies in recently published reports. The final columns of the two tables broadly categorise the types of evidence and professional arguments offered in the documents for justifying the recommendations. These categories are discussed below.

5.4 SOURCES OF EVIDENCE FOR RECOMMENDATIONS ON SERVICE PROVISION

5.4.1 Manpower and workload surveys

The colleges and societies have repeatedly conducted surveys of their members over the past two or three decades to assess existing patterns of manning services provided by the specialties. In obstetrics and gynaecology, for instance, a 1973 report contained recommendations based on a survey of six district hospitals in England and Scotland: a district with a population of 300,000 and 5,000 deliveries annually would typically have four consultants (a ratio of 1:1,250 deliveries). The most recent college report on obstetrics recommends that the ideal ratio of consultants to annual deliveries is 1:500. The British Cardiac Society has conducted a series of biennial manpower surveys since the late 1970s, the eighth being held in 1992, and data have often been collected on facilities in cardiology departments. The data have been used to inform the development of guidance on the provision of cardiac facilities (such as a recommendation of four coronary care beds per 100,000 population).

The data from the manpower surveys have been used over the years to inform the Colleges and societies in matters relating to (a) the regulation of consultant manpower and (b) policies that might affect traditional working patterns of consultant staff. Until the late 1980s the supply of NHS consultant posts in England was tightly regulated with annual guidelines being issued centrally on the estab-

Table 5.1 Recommendations made by Royal Colleges and specialist societies on patterns of consultant staffing for specialties in district hospitals

Specialties in district hospitals & year of reports	Recommendations for consultant staffing in district hospitals				
	Consultant/ population ratio	Size of consultant team in district hospital	Target population covered	Minimum workload annually	Justification for recommendations
General medicine (major specialities) 1993, 1994, 1996	1:50–100,000 for Cardiology, Diabetes & endocrinology, Gastroenterology, Respiratory, Renal medicine, Neurology Rheumatology	14	200–300,000	—	Manpower and workload surveys International comparisons Sub-specialist interests
Accident & emergency 1993	—	2 for 25–50,000 3 for 50–75,000 4 for 75–100,000 new patients annually	—	25,000 new patients for training	Workload survey Clinical quality
General surgery (1997 draft)	1:30,000	15 (At least 2 per major sub-speciality)	450–500,000	—	Clinical quality Sub-specialist interests
Trauma & orthopaedic surgery (1997 draft)	1:30–33,000	5–6	160,000	—	Manpower and workload surveys Clinical quality Sub-specialist interests
ENT surgery 1993	1:80,000	3	250,000	—	Expensive technology
Paediatrics 1996	—	5	—	(1800 admissions for training)	Manpower and workload surveys Clinical quality
Obstetrics 1994	—	1:500 deliveries annually	—	—	—
Clinical radiology 1995	—	8	300,000	12,500 exam-inations on average per consultant	Clinical quality Sub-specialist interests

Sources: Reports published by the medical Royal Colleges and specialist societies

lishment of new consultant posts in the various specialties. Evidence from the surveys was potentially useful for developing submissions in favour of expanding the consultant base of a specialty.

5.4.2 International comparisons

Various studies have demonstrated that trained specialist manpower levels in NHS hospitals in England and Wales are considerably lower than in most other countries in Western Europe and North America. The colleges and societies have, understandably, drawn on international comparisons for their respective specialties, usually in terms of population/ staffing ratios. Such international comparisons are unconvincing without careful examination of the reasons for differences in population/ staffing ratios, or workload. Such differences could be sensible adjustments to the incidence of conditions or relative input prices. Without such analysis they could equally well be used to support the argument that in other countries there are too many doctors per head of population seeing too few patients.

Table 5.2 Recommendations made by Royal Colleges and specialist societies on patterns of consultant staffing for specialties in regional or sub-regional centres

Specialties in regional/sub-regional centres & year of reports	Recommendations for consultant staffing in regional or sub-regional centres				
	Consultant/ population ratio	Size of consultant team in centre	Target population covered	Minimum workload annually	Justification for recommendations
Cardiology (angioplasty) 1996	—	2–3 trained operators	500,000 minimum	200 procedures (Target 400 procedures per million)	Clinical quality
Cardio-thoracic surgery 1992, 1994	—	3–4 cardiac 1–2 thoracic	1.5-2 million	800 cardiac operations 250 thoracic operations	Clinical quality
Urology 1993	1:100,000	6	600,000	—	Consultant-based service Expensive technology
Renal transplantation 1996 (draft)	—	—	2 million	50–60 transplants	Expensive support services
Clinical oncology in a cancer centre 1995, 1996	—	—	600,000	Maximum of 350 new patients per oncologist	International comparisons Clinical quality Access to pathology services
Paediatrics: Cardiology	1:1 million	3	2.5-3 million	—	Clinical quality
Cardiac surgery	—	2	2–3 million	—	Clinical quality
Diabetes & endocrinology	1:1,5–2 million	—	1.5 million	—	Clinical quality
Gastro-enterology	1:1 million	2–3	2–3 million	—	Clinical quality
Clinical genetics 1995	1:1 million	—	–	—	Clinical quality

Sources: Reports published by the medical Royal Colleges and specialist societies

5.4.3 Evidence on clinical quality

Medical audit, coupled with the development of clinical guidelines, was widely encouraged by the colleges in the late 1980s. But perhaps the most significant audit initiative was the launching of the independent national confidential enquiry into perioperative deaths (NCEPOD) in 1988, following a pilot enquiry conducted in three health regions. The enquiry is a continuous audit involving anaesthetists, gynaecologists and surgeons working in the NHS and independent hospitals in England, Wales, Northern Ireland, Jersey,

Guernsey and the Isle of Man. The fifth report was published in November 1996 (NCEPOD 1996). Data contained in the various reports on unsupervised clinical operations performed out of hours by doctors in training have undoubtedly influenced policy makers in the colleges and societies.

Ad hoc clinical audits have been commissioned occasionally by the colleges and societies. In 1986, a working party of the Royal College of Surgeons of England studied standards of care in the management of major injuries. Four independent assessors reviewed a thousand consecutive deaths from injury. A fifth of the deaths of patients admitted alive to hospital were judged by all assessors to have been potentially preventable (Anderson et al, 1988). Prompted by the findings, the Royal College formulated guidance for trauma services, including the recommendation on the availability of 24-hour CT scanning facilities for head injuries in A&E training departments. The British Orthopaedic Association later supplemented the head injury survey by a survey of fracture services in hospitals.

The systematic reviews to assess research into the possible relationship between volume of clinical activity and the quality of healthcare outcomes (see Chapter 2) established that most identified studies did not sufficiently take into account the effects of differences in patient case-mix. In the absence of such evidence, the Colleges and societies have had to rely on the research that is available. The field of cardiac care has a large body of international research literature, and so documents prepared by the cardiac societies tend to be comprehensively referenced. In general surgery, attention is now being focused on the output of a series of longitudinal audits being conducted in Scotland on large bowel cancer, breast cancer, and aortic aneurysms. These audits may be instructive with respect to the variables of case-mix and operator proficiency.

5.5 PROFESSIONAL JUSTIFICATION FOR RECOMMENDATIONS ON SERVICE PROVISION

5.5.1 Sub-specialist interests

Within most of the large specialties numerous sub-specialty groupings have been formed over the past decade or so. For example, paediatrics as a specialty encompasses 15 specialist areas, with the largest having their own associations. Some medical innovations have led to the blurring of historic boundaries between medical, surgical, anaesthetic and diagnostic specialties. This development, in turn, has fostered the formation of sub-specialty groupings with multi-disciplinary membership (in the field of gastroenterology, for example).

A paramount concern of the colleges and societies is that patients should be treated, when appropriate, by clinicians with suitable sub-specialist expertise. Moreover, doctors who practise as sub-specialists in district hospitals or regional centres should be regularly exposed to 'sufficient' quantities of relevant case material. High levels of exposure are considered necessary for sub-specialist training on the one hand, and for maintaining consultant proficiency on the other hand. This 'volume' argument helps to explain why the Senate of Surgery of Great Britain and Ireland is considering a proposal that the critical size of an acute hospital surgical service would be one serving a catchment population of 450,000–500,000, and the general surgical sub-specialties represented would be upper gastrointestinal, hepato-biliary, coloproctology, breast, endocrine, general paediatric, and vascular surgery.

Increased specialisation has implications for the organisation of services. Consider a situation in which it is felt that the d members of a specialty at a facility should see on average n patients of type s each year, either to maintain their skill level or to build up skills. Suppose that the proportion of patients of this type is p. Then this requires a flow of dn/p patients through the facility each year. Now suppose that technological developments mean that patients of type s can now be differentiated into two sub-types s_1 and s_2 occurring in proportions p_1 and p_2 in the population, where of course $p_1 + p_2 = p$. The two sub-types are seen by members of the sub-specialties formed from the original specialty. There are d_1 doctors in each sub-specialty where $d_1 + d_2 = d$. Then if each doctor in each sub-specialty needs to see on average n patients of the relevant type the required patient flow through the facility is the *maximum* of d_1n/p_1 and d_2n/p_2. This cannot be smaller than dn/p and will be larger unless the specialty divides into sub-specialties in exactly the same proportion as the sub-types of patients in the population. This seems unlikely to occur: some sub-types are more interesting to work with than others or have a better prognosis. An increase in the required patient flow may then require concentration of facilities.

There are other reasons why increasing sub-specialisation would tend to increase pressures for concentrating services. It can be argued that the maintenance of the skill and expertise of doctors requires them to have a certain minimum number of work-place colleagues in the same specialty. Hence increasing specialisation requires a larger number of doctors in one facility, and if the number of doctors is held constant this must imply fewer facilities. Increasing specialisation may also lead to doctors having to travel between sites to see a sufficient number of patients or to facilities being concentrated on one site.

5.5.2 Consultant-based versus consultant-led services

The concepts of 'consultant-based' and 'consultant-led' services have been introduced in certain specialties to distinguish between services in which consultants primarily undertake the clinical workload, and services which are heavily dependent on other grades of doctors to deliver care. A&E medicine is recognised within the specialty as being a consultant-led service. A&E departments in district hospitals receive high volumes of patients, the great majority being ambulatory and not requiring life-saving support or assessment for in-patient admission. The departments are typically staffed by two or three consultants and a team of doctors of intermediate and junior status. The greater proportion of the weekly caseloads are seen by the intermediate or junior medical staff. Some other specialties, which currently depend upon intermediate or junior staff for delivering services, aim to become consultant-based services and staffed accordingly. The society for urology, which has recommended that the services of its members are provided from sub-regional centres (Table 5.2), considers that urological surgery is a discipline that should be carried out as far as possible at consultant level partly because of the specialty's dependency on high technology.

Whilst the quality of patient care delivered by a consultant-based service should, in principle, be of the highest standard, the costs incurred by trusts of employing consultants in sufficient numbers to ensure that their duty rosters for emergency work are balanced by adequate off-duty periods could prove prohibitive. Furthermore, over the next few years there is likely to be an insufficient supply in many specialties of fully trained doctors for appointment to new consultant posts in expanding departments. Paediatrics already has a relatively high number of consultant posts that are either unfilled or filled by locum appointments. In clinical radiology, likewise, there is currently a substantial imbalance between vacancies for consultant appointments and numbers of doctors attaining CCST.

5.5.3 Emergency surgical services

An administrative reason for recommending that surgical services would best be provided from units serving catchment populations of 450,000–500,000 is that emergency surgical care would be more easily organised. More importantly, from the patients' perspective, it is suggested that the quality of emergency care would be improved. The volume of emergency work would justify the provision of a dedicated 24-hour emergency theatre. Emergency rotas for consultant teams would be better organised. In general surgery, for example, emergency rota duties would be no more frequent than one in five, and during each 24-hour weekday period, when a consultant team was 'on take', routinely scheduled operating lists would not be done by team members. Senior team members would be available instead to assess clinically patients referred with acute conditions, thus reducing the likelihood of cases being admitted or operated on inappropriately.

5.5.4 Centralisation of expensive technology

Otorhinolaryngology (ENT surgery) and urology are two specialties requiring the use of expensive facilities (equipment and imaging techniques) to provide modern treatments. The societies for these specialties consider that the costs of equipping services will promote centralisation.

5.5.5 Access to laboratory and radiological services

Laboratory and radiological services are an integral part of clinical services and play a key role in their delivery. At the present time the delivery of cancer care is receiving special attention. Cancer centres are likely to become the 'hubs' of networks of cancer services in Britain. From the perspective of clinical oncology, the arrangements will be strengthened if the centres are served by departments of pathology with sufficient expertise to provide tumour panels of pathologists, clinical radiology departments with access to the full range of modern diagnostic techniques, and other specialist and diagnostic services. With renal transplantation, avoidance of duplicating specialised resources (such as tissue-typing laboratories that provide 24-hour services and organ retrieval teams) has been offered as a justification for centralising transplantation services.

5.6 ISSUES RAISED BY THE RECOMMENDATIONS

5.6.1 Implications for other aspects of the service

The annual flow of patients through a facility (whether a hospital or a hospital department) has implications for a number of important aspects of the service provided, in addition to its impact on training and skill maintenance. Consideration of the different aspects may imply different recommendations for patient flow. The different aspects interact and determining the optimal throughput of a facility will require examination of the system-wide effects.

Hospital costs. The costs per case incurred by a hospital initially fall with patient throughput, remain constant over a fairly wide range and then increase. The range of throughput over which unit cost is minimised varies across different specialties. A concern only with hospital costs would require throughput to fall in the flat portion of the average cost curve.

Competition. More throughput, other things

equal, implies fewer but larger facilities and hence less potential competition between them for patients. The welfare implications depend on how hospital behaviour and performance is affected by the number and size of hospitals in the market for hospital care. More competition might mean greater incentives for efficiency within hospitals. It might lead to lower prices for care. If purchasers respond to lower prices by increasing demand the number of cases treated will increase, thus benefiting patients who would not otherwise have been treated and lowering the waiting times for all patients. If demand does not respond reductions in prices merely redistribute funds towards purchasers and the welfare consequences depend on how the funds are spent.

The marginal impact of numbers of competitors on the degree of competition in a market is likely to diminish fairly rapidly though different economic models provide different answers to the question of 'How rapidly?'.

Quality of care. The evidence elsewhere in this volume suggests that quality of care, at least as conventionally measured, increases initially with patient throughput but that after fairly small throughput levels are achieved, the marginal improvements in quality are zero.

Other public sector costs. If an increase in patient throughput, other things being equal, implies fewer facilities this will have an impact on costs incurred outside the facilities. The most obvious example is that with fewer, and therefore more widely dispersed, facilities ambulance costs will increase. Ambulance service costs per case will increase as the number of facilities falls and will do so at an increasing rate because the distance that patients have to be transported will increase more rapidly the fewer the number of facilities.

Private sector costs. The number of facilities will also have implications for patients and their families. Fewer, more widely dispersed facilities, will increase the access costs for patients and, like ambulance costs, these costs increase more rapidly the fewer the facilities available. A concern only with patient access costs would imply that there should be more rather than fewer facilities.

5.6.2 Interactions: the service as a system

Evaluation of recommendations for changes in required throughput for training or skill maintenance purposes needs to take account of the fact that the NHS is a system: changes in one aspect will have repercussions for other aspects. This is not just because throughput has implications for costs, quality, patient accessibility, etc., but because these interact. Amalgamating existing facilities on one site to generate a given throughput will affect the costs borne by patients. Increased access costs will reduce the flow of patients from a given population. This may change costs elsewhere in the system, for example, by altering the workload in general practice. It may also alter the mix of patients seen in the facility. The reduced demand from the population and the change in patient-mix may in turn affect the patient flow requirements. Changes in the mix of patients will have implications for unit costs for any given throughput.

Two of these factors (patient access and ambulance service costs) imply dispersed facilities, whilst the evidence in other chapters suggests that the other two factors of training and skill maintenance imply more concentrated configurations, with unit cost minimization requiring somewhat larger levels of throughput than quality maximisation. The choice of service configuration should therefore balance its implications for these access factors as well as its implications for skill acquisition and maintenance. The overall optimal configuration will not be ideal from the point of view of any of these aspects. To choose the optimal configuration we need to be able to specify the relationship between configuration and each of the factors and the relative weights to be given to the factors. In short we must recognise that decisions about service configuration embody tradeoffs. It will not be easy to decide whether, say, possible benefits from concentration in services are worth the reduction in ease of access for patients, but such judgements are better made explicitly so that the implied valuations and the quality of the evidence can be examined.

Whilst there is evidence on, and models of, the relationship between costs, quality and accessibility, the picture as regards skill acquisition and maintenance is much murkier. The ultimate reason for being concerned about the stock of skills and experience in the workforce (its human capital) is because of the effect of increases in human capital on the quality and cost-effectiveness of care provided to patients. To make rational decisions about whether it is worthwhile changing the configuration of the service to improve the human capital of the workforce we need to be able to estimate the effects of greater skill and experience on the quality of care. The evidence from the NCEPOD studies (NCEPOD, 1996) indicates, unsurprisingly, that more senior doctors provide better quality care. The evidence available does not yet enable one to estimate the relationship between quality of care and level of experience. We do not know how rapidly the stock of skill increases with the flow of patients seen, nor how rapidly that stock depreciates. In short, the marginal value of additional throughput in increasing and maintaining skill is not known.

Nor is there any very clear specification of what is meant by 'experience'. Most of the skill-related requirements for service configuration are expressed in terms of a throughput of patients. Increased throughput could be valuable for two reasons: greater experience of particular types of case and experience of a wider range of cases. These could have very different implications for the required increase in throughput.

5.6.3 What are the policy margins?

An increase in experience can be achieved in a variety of ways of which increased throughput is one. Increases in patient throughput can be achieved by concentrating facilities with length of stay remaining constant or by reducing length of stay. Concentration of facilities will increase patient access costs and change the mix of patients seen. Increasing throughput in a given facility by reducing length of stay will also change the experience of doctors since patients of a given type will stay for less time.

Increased throughput from a given population will also change the mix of patients admitted.

Distance-learning courses and audio-visual, computer-aided instruction packages can be used to enhance skills and experience from a given service configuration. Courses and learning aids also have smaller costs in terms of the other factors which need to be taken into account when choosing a service configuration.

5.7 CONCLUSIONS

Service recommendations of the Royal Colleges and specialist societies are purely advisory and cannot be enforced in any formal sense. These recommendations may nonetheless have an impact on service configuration. To the extent that purchasers use Royal College and other authoritative sources of guidance in drafting contracts, service recommendations may act as a constraint on the behaviour of provider units. The requirements of the Royal Colleges and higher training committees for training recognition are of greater direct relevance for concentration: partly because these recommendations can be enforced, and partly because loss of training recognition will make it more difficult for a trust to staff a service adequately.

From a health service management standpoint, there is a perception in trusts and health authorities that the Royal Colleges tend to be reactive rather than proactive, although it is recognised that they have an important role to play in many areas, including the promotion of new developments and maintaining standards of care (YHEC, 1996). Over the next few years significant changes will be observed in the staffing of hospital medical services as a consequence of the fully implemented New Deal arrangements and the reformed system for higher specialist training. But these changes were brought about by Government policies, and the Colleges' role has been to inform the decision making and to act as independent authorities for monitoring the system of post-graduate training.

The reports on service matters from the Colleges and specialist societies have fre-

quently contained recommendations on staffing clinical services, usually expressed as simple population/manpower ratios. The ratios have invariably been lower than current practice (often a lot lower). But in the absence of adequate supporting evidence, it has not been possible for readers to assess whether the recommended ratios were fully justifiable. It is also the case that there has been very little systematic evidence available on relationships between process and outcome for differing service configurations within specialties.

There are two issues about which the Colleges and societies are particularly concerned at present: sub-specialisation and the delivery of emergency care. On the one hand, the acquisition and maintenance of sub-specialist skills is presented as a strong argument for concentrating services; but at the same time, there are anxieties that by concentrating services, access to emergency care may be restricted in certain localities or for selected patient groups (Royal College of Physicians, 1996).

There are pressures now for obtaining concerted guidance on these issues. In April 1997, the NHS Executive issued for consultation a working draft from which to develop a 'quality framework' for hospital medical and dental staffing (NHS Executive, 1997). It is intended that the framework become a key strand of a new medical workforce strategy based on quality. The framework will provide the context for local medical workforce advisory groups (LMWAGS), which were set up regionally in 1996 to comment and advise on current and future medical staffing plans of individual trusts as set out in their strategic and annual business plans. The working draft suggests that LMWAGS first consider medical staffing profiles in trusts, particularly for specialties in trusts which fall into the lowest 10 per cent of the distribution nationally. Baseline medical staffing ratios are provided in the working draft, but they relate only to (a) categories of medical staff (consultants, 'juniors', other career grades); (b) types of trusts (e.g. acute hospital, acute mixed, acute teaching, community mental health) and (c) broad specialty groupings. The document does not offer guidance on how LMWAGS might integrate data on staffing levels with information relating to training and skill maintenance that needs to be taken into account when determining optimal staffing configurations for local services.

The prevailing message from this volume is that only a scanty evidence base exists for informing the development of policies and guidance on centralisation with respect to training and skill maintenance. Moreover, any deliberations need to accept that the NHS is a system and changes effected in one aspect (e.g. in hospital facilities) will have repercussions for other aspects: by possibly increasing workloads in primary care or demands on ambulance services or restricting access for patients. Even within a hospital facility, changing the configuration of a specialty's service could result in altered patterns of throughput, case-mix, and average lengths of stay, and these might have a deleterious effect on training instead of an anticipated benefit.

Because of the dynamism of the health service as a system, the arguments for greater concentration of facilities to improve skill acquisition and maintenance need to be treated with considerable caution for the time being. There is clearly a need for conceptual modelling to be undertaken and appropriate evidence collected for analysing the models. This would be a considerable task requiring multiprofessional input, but one which could be successfully performed by medical Royal Colleges working together with academics drawn from different disciplines (e.g. economics, operational research, public health), postgraduate educationalists and representatives of NHS purchasers and providers.

REFERENCES

Anderson I D, Woodford M, de Dombal F T, Irving M 1988 Retrospective Study of 1000 Deaths from Injury in England and Wales. British Medical Journal, vol 296, 1305–8.

Department of Health 1993 Hospital Doctors: Training for the Future. The Report of the Working Group on Specialist Medical Training (chairman Dr Kenneth Calman). Department of Health, London.

Department of Health 1996a Health and Personal Social Services Statistics for England. 1996 edition. The Stationery Office, London.

Department of Health 1996b Hospital, Public Health Medicine and Community Health Service Medical and Dental Staff in England 1985 to 1995. Statistical Bulletin 1996/18.

Dowie R 1990 Patterns of Hospital Medical Staffing: Junior Doctors' Hours. British Postgraduate Medical Federation, London.

National Confidential Enquiry into Perioperative Deaths 1996 The Report of the National Confidential Enquiry into Perioperative Deaths 1993/1994. NCEPOD, London.

NHS Executive 1996 Funding PGMDE. A Review of the EL(92) 63 Arrangements for Funding Postgraduate Medical and Dental Education in England. Report of the Steering Group. Department of Health, Leeds.

NHS Executive 1997 A Working Draft to Develop the Quality Framework for HCHS Medical & Dental Staffing. NHS Executive, Leeds.

NHS Management Executive 1991a Junior Doctors: the New Deal. (Information pack.) Department of Health, London.

NHS Management Executive 1991b Working for Patients. Postgraduate and Continuing Medical and Dental Education. Department of Health, London.

Royal College of Physicians 1996 Future Patterns of Care by General and Specialist Physicians. Royal College of Physicians of London, London.

Stern M, Brennan S (no date) Medical Audit in the Hospital and Community Health Service. Department of Health, Wetherby.

York Health Economics Consortium 1996 Concentration and Choice in the Provision of Hospital Services. Content of Recommendations of Royal Colleges and Professional Associations and their Implications for Configuration of Services. Technical Appendix 4, volumes I & II. University of York, York.

6

The case for and against mergers

Brian Ferguson, Maria Goddard

6.1 INTRODUCTION

A central theme of the NHS reforms was the introduction of supply-side competition. Hospital Trusts would compete with each other to win contracts from purchasers, leading to improved efficiency and responsiveness in the delivery of healthcare services. Although it was recognised that the scope for competition would vary geographically and with different types of services, the Government reiterated the importance of the role of provider competition more recently in the guidance issued on mergers and joint ventures (NHS Executive, 1994). This emphasised the need to consider the impact of mergers between hospitals or individual services on the level of competition in the relevant market, stating that such developments should only go ahead where the benefits from merger would outweigh any anti-competitive effects.

However, despite this emphasis on competition, several commentators have noted the trend towards concentration of services in the NHS (Harrison and Prentice, 1996; NAHAT, 1994) and there has been speculation that the number of hospitals will fall dramatically. Indeed, *The Independent* (24 March 1997) reported the Labour Party's intention to view hospital mergers as a means of achieving significant healthcare cost savings. In contrast, other policies have suggested a commitment to small local hospitals, emphasising their important role in the provision of NHS care (NHS Executive Press Release, 8 January 1996), so there appear to be forces pulling in opposite directions. Although the concentration of hospital services is often assumed to be a good thing because of perceived efficiency gains and quality improvements, the supporting evidence for such gains is not definitive. There are also trade-offs to be made in terms of patient choice and accessibility (see Chapter 4).

The economic rationale underlying mergers in the healthcare sector is considered in this Chapter, alongside relevant evidence for and against further concentration arising from this route. Much depends upon the reasons for merger of particular services or hospitals, hence these are discussed in detail. Also reported is a survey of NHS Regional Offices to explore some of the conceptual issues using examples of mergers which have actually taken place or are being proposed.

6.2 WHAT IS MEANT BY 'MERGER'?

Mergers can take a variety of forms. In other sectors vertical mergers involve the combination of firms at different stages of the production process, with a single firm producing the goods or services that either suppliers or customers could provide. Horizontal mergers involve the combination of two or more firms producing similar goods or services. There is also a distinction between merger and consolidation as the former technically refers to the dissolution of one or more organisations and their assimilation by another (this arrangement can also be classed as an acquisition if the status of each party is unequal and depending on the arrangements for purchase); the latter involves the formation of a new organisation following the dissolution of two or more organisations. The term 'merger' is used in this chapter to cover both consolidation and merger as defined above.

In the healthcare sector it is common to use the term 'integration' rather than merger to represent the various restructuring activities which, in some countries, are seen to be contributing towards the development of seamless care. The type of arrangements between organisations involved in such cases varies enormously, but the most vital distinction in terms of the discussion of merger is the extent to which the alliances, partnerships, joint operating arrangements and other co-operative arrangements rely on contractual (in the form of either short or long-term contracts) relationships rather than the unified ownership or management of the integrated parties which characterise mergers. It is often the case that joint ventures and similar arrangements lead eventually to merger between the two parties, and this has led the former to be characterised as 'dating' with the merger as 'marriage' (Lazarus, 1995). As discussed later, arrangements which fall short of actual merger may be potentially more important in terms of their effect on the healthcare market than formal mergers.

The discussion in this Chapter centres around horizontal rather than vertical mergers, although the latter are becoming more important in some areas. For example, in the USA, there is some evidence to suggest that hospitals are developing their own health insurance plans (such as HMOs), but the extent to which this vertical integration is successful depends on the reaction of competing HMOs, which may threaten to stop using the provider if their HMO suffers (Miller, 1996). Health plans and insurers are already involved in acquiring their healthcare providers in some areas (e.g. Kaiser). Hospitals are also attempting greater integration with physicians through a variety of management services organisations or acquisition (Miller, 1996). In the UK, GP fundholders increasingly resemble vertically integrated units as they are able to supply in-house some of the services (e.g. minor operations) which they formerly purchased from other healthcare providers, saving some of their funds for alternative uses.

Mergers may occur within a single geographical market or across markets. Horizontal mergers across geographical markets as in the development of hospital chains in the USA are often seen as posing fewer problems for antitrust policy as long as their share of local markets remains at an acceptable level. Indeed, as the greatest threat of entry to a local market may come not from alternative local providers but from national and regional chains outside the local market, it could be argued that this promotes rather than hinders competition and contestability (Robinson and Casalino, 1996). In the UK there has been some speculation about the development of ownership chains, but proposals by Trusts to set up *new* sites in other areas may be outside the current law (Health Services Journal, 4 August 1994), although the management of existing sites may be feasible.

A further distinction is necessary in the discussion of mergers in the NHS: mergers at the Trust level and at the level of individual services. Mergers between whole Trusts are not as common as the merger of services or specialties currently provided at more than one location on a single site. The latter has no impact on competition if the sites are owned by the same Trust, but where there is an arrangement to relocate services at one Trust rather than two or more, competition for that service may indeed be affected. The importance of this sort of reconfiguration which falls short of merger is acknowledged in the guidance issued by the Department of Health, which covers not only formal mergers but also merger activity involving services or specialties (NHS Executive, 1994).

6.3 THE ECONOMIC RATIONALE FOR MERGERS

6.3.1 The general case

Horizontal merger is one route through which a firm can acquire dominance over the supply of goods or services in a market. A dominant or monopolistic supplier may have the ability to restrict the volume of service or charge higher prices than would prevail in a more competitive environment, resulting in a loss of welfare (Vickers and Hay, 1987). The internal efficiency of the firm may also depend in part on the degree of competition faced by the decision-makers within the firm. A dominant firm will face poor incentives to achieve productive efficiency and its key decision-makers may seek above all a quiet life, with a tendency to be slow to innovate (Vita et al, 1991). Balanced against this is the need to consider the possible efficiency gains from merger, which should be weighed against increases in market power, reflecting a welfare trade-off approach to merger (Mueller, 1996).

Although merger is one route through which market power can be created, market concen-

tration and market power are by no means equivalent. The extent to which a dominant firm can maintain a price higher than the competitive level will also depend upon the responsiveness of customers and other suppliers to changes in relative prices. This will depend not only on market share but also on factors such as the availability of substitutes for the product, the level of spare capacity and ease of entry to the market.

In markets where there are sufficient competitors to prevent the emergence of a single dominant firm, collusive behaviour may still be an issue. If merger activity creates a small number of relatively large firms within a market, there is a possibility that they will co-operate in order to produce non-competitive outcomes. Certain market conditions will increase the likelihood of collusive agreements and explicit or tacit cartels, mainly relating to the type of information which participants can gain about their rivals and their actions (Vita et al, 1991). The extent to which collusion can allow abuse of market power will again depend upon the responsiveness of demand to price changes, and on the behaviour of firms in terms of how they expect rivals to react to unilateral price changes (Ferguson and Posnett, 1994).

6.3.2 The healthcare sector

To what extent are mergers, as one route to acquiring monopoly power, a potential cause for concern in the healthcare system? Clearly they are considered important by some governments which have set out how their general policy on mergers applies to the hospital sector. In the USA, policy governing horizontal mergers has been applied to the hospital sector (Department of Justice/Federal Trade Commission, 1992); in the UK, the mergers and joint ventures guidance is more recent (NHS Executive, 1994).

Some would argue about the relevance of analysing healthcare markets using an economic framework based on traditional monopoly theory, pointing particularly to the nature of institutions and relationships in the NHS which suggests that competitive behaviour is either not possible or may be inefficient (Craig and Forbes, 1996; Dawson, 1995). However, acknowledging the special nature of the market participants in the NHS and the fact that perfectly competitive markets rarely exist, does not mean that monopoly power is an issue which can safely be ignored.

First, there may be weak incentives for monopoly providers to operate at minimum cost: that is, to achieve productive efficiency. Implementing cost-saving mechanisms is likely to cause Trust management considerable time and effort, so avoiding such practices is likely to be attractive to Trusts enjoying a degree of market power. Second, the pricing regime in the NHS, which allows Trusts to cover costs plus an allowance for rate of return on capital, provides even more incentives for those in monopoly positions to put less effort into reducing costs as they are easily able to pass cost increases directly onto purchasers in the form of higher prices.

Where providers enjoy a dominant position for some services and not others, they have an incentive to load higher proportions of fixed costs onto those services in which they have a monopoly whilst pricing other services more competitively. Although in theory such planned cross-subsidisation is not allowed, in practice there may well be scope to engage in such activities as accounting practices are not sophisticated enough to allow detection. Unless it is argued that price has absolutely no impact on purchasing decisions, then policies which help to discourage this activity will be potentially beneficial. This is actually reflected in the USA policy emphasis on the extent to which post-merger market structure is likely to encourage subsequent efficiency-enhancing efforts, where it is noted that this is a particular problem in the case of non-profit hospitals, which have less incentive to reduce costs in order to reap larger profits (Vistnes, 1995). In addition, this may be reflected not only in cost-reducing efforts but also in terms of lower quality and a lack of responsiveness and innovation in services.

The extent to which a dominant provider can exercise market power in the NHS is likely to vary considerably between services. For those services where purchasers can shift some or all of their business, as patients are more willing to travel, and where alternative providers may find it relatively easy to enter the market, even a dominant hospital would find it difficult to maintain high prices and/or poor quality over time. This may be true for some elective services but it is unlikely to be the case for services such as emergency care, where providers are more easily able to take advantage of their dominance owing to lack of potential entrants and the importance of easy access. In such cases, contestability (the threat of competition) rather than actual competition will be the relevant issue.

Although quantitative evidence is not available, some purchasers attribute their success in achieving gains from the reformed NHS to their ability to switch business between providers, even if this concerns a relatively small proportion of overall business (Redmayne, 1995, 1996). Indeed, even where geographical circumstances will not permit competition in the market, some purchasers have realised that their future leverage with providers depends upon the creation of contestability (e.g. Redmayne, 1996, p41). Hence it is important that providers who gain market power through merger still perceive the *threat* of competition, even if the existing degree of competition is relatively low.

6.4 TRENDS IN MERGER ACTIVITY IN THE HEALTHCARE SECTOR

Mergers between NHS Trusts are recorded by the Department of Health, where they require ministerial approval. Since 1991, thirteen mergers have been approved and undertaken; one has been approved and commenced in April 1997; and consultation is currently underway for several more (NHS Executive, personal communication, December 1996). The mergers differ in nature with some involving community and mental-health services (e.g. West Dorset); others involving acute and community mergers (e.g. Isle of Wight Community and St Mary's Acute); whilst others join together larger acute Trusts (e.g. Guys and St Thomas). At the time of writing, consultation is taking place on substantial acute hospital mergers in the cities of Leeds and Newcastle upon Tyne. These figures underestimate the true extent of merger activity in the NHS for two reasons.

First, those which do not involve the dissolution of one Trust as part of the merger process do not require Ministerial approval so are not included. Thus the 'take-over' of smaller units by an established Trust will not appear (e.g. merger between Premier Health Trust in the West Midlands and five small acute hospitals). Neither will those mergers which occurred at the early stages of the reforms where a first or second wave Trust took over an existing Directly Managed Unit (DMU) (e.g. Northgate Trust with Prudhoe DMU in Northern and Yorkshire; Birmingham Heartlands with Solihull Hospital DMU).

Second, merger activity below the level of the whole Trust which may involve significant reconfiguration and concentration will not appear as they do not count as official mergers. The importance of such developments is acknowledged in the Department of Health's guidance on mergers, but no formal record of these changes is kept, making it difficult to draw an overall picture of how service concentration has changed. However, acute-service reviews have been undertaken in almost every city and in many this has led to increased service concentration (Turner, 1994 and 1995). A recent review of acute service reconfigurations in twenty commissioning authorities reinforces the overall picture of increased concentration in services and specialties (Turner, 1996).

Although increased concentration in the form of fewer and larger hospitals is not wholly attributable to merger activity, data showing the growth of larger hospitals (apart from those in the >1000 beds group) and the reduction in smaller hospitals can be revealing (see Table 6.1).

Table 6.1 Proportion of non-psychiatric hospitals by size, England

Size (no. of beds)	1959	1979	1989/90
<50	42.7%	37.4%	35.5%
51–250	43.3%	43.8%	41.8%
251–500	10.1%	11.8%	13.7%
501–1,000	3.6%	6.4%	8.9%
>1,000	0.4%	0.6%	0.3%

Source: adapted from Harrison and Prentice (1996)

Significant merger activity appears likely to continue in the NHS, especially as almost every health authority and region is undertaking some sort of review of acute services provision. Indeed, the review of acute services in Leeds concluded with a strong recommendation from the review team for a merger between St James and Seacroft Trust and United Leeds Hospitals Trust, potentially creating the largest Trust in the country (Leeds Review Task Force, 1996). Similarly, a review of acute Trusts in Oxfordshire considered the need to reduce the number of Trusts from eight to around four (Oxfordshire Health Authority, December 1996). Media reports constantly refer to proposals for new mergers or rumours about mergers in the pipeline (e.g. HSJ, 11 July 1996; 18 July 1996 a and b; 15 August 1996; 31 October, 1996; 23 January 1997a).

6.5 WHY DO HOSPITALS MERGE?

The theory of the dominant firm would predict that one reason for merger activity is the desire to acquire market power and take advantage of a monopoly position. However, whilst the creation of a dominant provider which can exercise market power may well be one *consequence* of mergers between hospitals, there is some evidence which suggests there may be more important drivers for merger other than the desire to exploit monopoly power. This may be especially true for NHS Trusts which do not have a strong profit-making incentive.

6.5.1 Removal of excess capacity

In the early years of the reforms, many of the reconfigurations in the hospital sector were said to be due to the existence of spare capacity in the acute sector which needed to be dealt with in a planned way rather than being left to the market. For example, the reconfigurations brought about by the Tomlinson report on hospital services in London arose as a result of a perceived mismatch between over-supply of secondary care (estimated to be between 1,365 and 7,200 "excess beds") and under-supply of good quality primary care (Tomlinson, 1992; Department of Health, 1993).

Where genuine over-supply exists and fixed resources are being under-utilised, mergers can produce short-run cash savings and reduce average costs through better utilisation of resources and avoiding duplication. It is, however, problematic to define 'over-supply', and in the UK this has led to debates about the number of beds required to meet demand. The NHS has witnessed a consistent decline in the total number of hospital beds available since 1984, as illustrated in Table 6.2.

At the same time, the demand for hospital services as measured by finished consultant episodes has risen, and over one million people remain on waiting lists. In addition, there has been an acceleration in emergency admissions, the causes of which are still being debated. Increased activity rates have been accommodated by much more intensive use of acute beds, shorter lengths of stay and a significant increase in day case activity (see Table 6.3).

The issue now appears to be whether there is still spare capacity in the acute sector which may lead to future merger activity, or whether some sort of critical level has been reached beyond which further reductions are not possible. This is not an easy question to answer and the use of bed norms per thousand population is no longer particularly relevant given changes in the nature of medical technology and healthcare provision. Whilst some would argue that the reduction in spare capacity has gone too far too quickly without a commensurate expansion of primary care (e.g. Jarman, 1993), and many Trusts are now struggling to meet demand at peak periods, there may still be specific geographical areas in which the reduction of acute spare capacity has driven reconfigurations and mergers. This has been especially true of large urban conurbations served by a number of general hospitals, all of which could not be sustained in their original

forms in the face of the shifting emphasis to primary care.

In conclusion, whilst it may be the case that specific geographical areas still face a degree of spare capacity which merger could potentially eliminate, it is clear that there has already been a substantial reduction in apparent excess capacity in the acute sector and it is not clear how much scope there is for this to continue. Moreover, as the greatest resource savings will accrue where under-utilised capital is removed from the system following merger (both short-term cash gains and lower costs due to reduction in capital charges), those which do not result in the closure of hospital sites will not realise such gains. Given the political and public emphasis on retaining access to local hospitals despite mergers aimed at consolidating services (e.g. Solihull and Heartlands hospital merger in the West Midlands), it is possible that many mergers will fail to reap all the savings that might be predicted.

6.5.2 Economies of scale and scope

Distinct from the savings brought about by combining hospitals where each is experiencing excess capacity which can be eliminated through increasing activity, economies of scale refer to the benefits that can be achieved by operating efficiently at higher levels of production. If these exist, mergers which combine two efficient smaller hospitals into a single larger unit will reap efficiency gains. What is often overlooked is that empirical work on this issue assumes that hospitals are currently working efficiently, so the extent to which it can guide decisions on mergers involving hospitals which are not doing so is rather limited (Effective Health Care Bulletin, 1996).

Nevertheless, the claim that mergers will result in economies of scale, which will in turn

Table 6.2 Average number of available daily inpatient beds in all specialties (England)

	1984	1989/90	1990/91	1991/92	1992/93	1993/94	1994/95
Number of beds (000s)	335	270	255	243	232	219	212
Rate per 000 population	7.1	5.7	5.3	5.0	4.8	4.5	4.3

Source: Health and Personal Social Services Statistics (1996)

Table 6.3 Cases treated in all specialties (England)

	1984	1989/90	1990/91	1991/92	1992/93	1993/94	1994/95
In-patients (000s)	6,867	7,477	7,524	7,755	7,828	7,988	8,065
Day cases (000s)	903	1,163	1261	1,547	1,808	2,106	2,474

Source: Health and Personal Social Services Statistics (1996)

produce efficiency gains, is a common argument and is reflected in the UK policy guidelines which include a summary of the evidence for the existence of both economies of scale and scope (NHS Executive, 1994, Appendix 1). One US study found that the achievement of economies of scale was cited frequently by merging parties as a main reason for merger (Greene, 1992).

Economies of scale and scope can be analysed in relation to both cost savings and quality gains. Whilst the arguments relating to a negative relationship between long-run average costs and the *volume* of production (economies of scale related to costs) is perhaps best known, the link between the *range* of services provided and costs (economies of scope in relation to costs) may be more pertinent to the provision of hospital care. As the treatment of a particular condition often requires an input from several specialties, it can be argued that having each specialty on one site will reduce costs. The desire to maintain or create links between specialties has indeed been offered as one reason for merger (Haggard, 1995). In addition, this has been a powerful argument in the debate about the number and configuration of A&E departments in the UK, where perceived links between specialties are an important consideration.

In relation to quality, the arguments for mergers producing economies of scope again appear superficially strong. The emphasis on seamless care for the patient and the benefits of having on a single site the full range of services which might be required for treatment have been used as a reason not only for the merger of whole hospitals, but also for the realignment of services between Trusts. For example, in the Leeds Acute Services Review, the argument for centralising many services on a single site was to ensure the availability of

specialties with 'critical links' to each other (Leeds Review Task Force, 1996). The arguments about a link between volume and quality (economies of scale in relation to quality) have been put forward in most of the major reconfigurations which have involved a greater concentration of services (Turner, 1996).

The evidence on economies of scale and scope was discussed in far greater detail in Chapter 3. For now, it is important to recognise that a belief in the existence of such economies remains a significant driving force behind many mergers, especially those at the specialty or service level.

6.5.3 INFLUENCE OF PROFESSIONAL GUIDANCE ON SERVICE DELIVERY

The importance of a perceived relationship between volume or range of services and quality of care has been enhanced by the views of various professional groups which often put forward guidance on the organisation of service delivery. This may take the form of guidance on the composition of the clinical team, the minimum population to be served or links between different professionals and specialties within the unit. For example, the British Paediatric Association has published recommendations on the care of critically ill children (BPA, 1993) which have implications for the minimum size of a unit and the range of services required to ensure good quality care. Whilst these may be disputed by some commentators on the grounds of lack of good research evidence and reliance on expert opinion (NHS Centre for Reviews and Dissemination, 1995), they remain influential in guiding purchasers' service specifications and in terms of the ability of Trusts to attract staff willing to work in units which do not conform to these standards.

A range of Royal College and other professional guidance for various specialties was reviewed and the results published in a report which also included the outcome of interviews with representatives from these organisations and senior managers from both Trusts and Health Authorities (YHEC, 1996). The authors found that very few guidance documents on service delivery cited published or unpublished literature in support of quality claims. However, a combination of minimum staffing numbers and consultant:population ratios, based largely on belief, led to recommendations for a minimum acceptable population to be served by all the main specialties. For more specialised services such as renal transplantation and coronary angioplasty, these recommendations are exerting pressure for concentration.

Whilst the guidance is just that – guidance – there is evidence to suggest that clinicians and managers consider these to be strong drivers towards concentration and hence merger (e.g. Turner, 1996).

6.5.4 Changes in training of medical staff

The above survey revealed that many NHS managers considered policy changes relating to training to be more influential than the service-delivery guidance in creating pressures to merge. First, the Royal Colleges again play an influential role as they set out the requirements which a hospital must meet in order to achieve training accreditation. If these are not met to the satisfaction of the relevant College (and there is some discretion in how they are applied), the hospital will find it almost impossible to attract junior doctors (who will be reluctant to spend time in a hospital without it counting towards training requirements) and thus it will be difficult to provide a service at all.

The training requirements relate to areas such as the minimum size of the unit in which the trainees work, the composition of their workload in terms of the number and range of cases they see, consultant staffing levels and supervision, specified time set aside for training, and resources available (such as library facilities). The emphasis on the quantity and range of cases seen suggests a relationship between workload and training outcomes, for which no evidence is cited nor found, being based instead on professional opinion and experience (YHEC, 1996).

The main driver to concentration results not just from the training requirements but from their interaction with the national policy of reduced hours of working for junior doctors (the 'New Deal' reforms). As the number of working hours permitted declines, then the number of trainees required to provide the same service will increase and each of these will be able to see fewer cases during the training period. The implications of this are twofold. First, the organisation of on-call rotas will be made more difficult as junior doctors play a major role in staffing these; second, doctors will be able to see fewer cases during their working hours than previously. If training requirements remain unchanged, larger volumes of service will be necessary in order to meet the minimum workload levels. Smaller departments which do not meet these levels may view merger with a department from another Trust as one option to overcome this problem and to avoid having to stop providing the service altogether (e.g. Health Service Journal, 3 August 1995; 18 July 1996). Purchasers may encourage such developments in order to ensure they have access to the service in a particular geographical area. The Leeds Review provides a good example of how staffing and training requirements appear to drive merger proposals between sites in specialties such as paediatric surgery, vascular surgery, ENT and urology (Leeds Acute Services Review, 1996).

Other national policies related to medical training are also likely to cause pressure for greater concentration of services and thus potential mergers at the specialty level. In particular, the reforms to specialist medical training which have recently been introduced (Calman, 1993) may affect the viability of small departments or small hospitals to continue to be accredited for training and thus make their future uncertain unless they combine into larger units. This is largely because the reforms will reduce the length of the training period, as well as requiring greater supervision from consultants, together with a reduction in the amount of time which junior doctors spend contributing towards service provision.

6.5.5 Government policy on service delivery

In some specific areas, Government policy outlines the way in which services are to be provided by proposing the requirements for a good service. One example of this is the Calman reforms on the provision of cancer services (Department of Health, 1995). Although the 'Calman Report' highlights the need for networks of expertise with primary care as the focus of care, it also calls for the creation of designated Cancer Units and Cancer Centres. A natural response of Trusts is to form alliances to put together a case for designated Cancer Unit status, covering an explicit range of cancer sites. There are several drivers underlying this, not least the belief that economies of scale will be achieved by concentrating activity. Also, the trend towards greater specialisation (even within particular types of cancer) is likely to lead to pressures to concentrate services, particularly if there is supporting evidence on a positive relationship between volume and quality. Such drivers will almost certainly increase the pressure to concentrate expertise, despite the underlying philosophy of the Calman Report, which is to take services to the patient. Reconfigurations of services, possibly involving Trust mergers or simply joint agreements to seek Cancer Unit or Centre status, will continue to take place to realise the perceived benefits of specialised cancer care.

6.5.6 Rescue of a failing Trust

There are a number of reasons why a Trust might no longer be financially viable and therefore merge with another Trust. For example, where there is excess capacity due to falling demand for hospital services, merger may be seen as a more palatable alternative to closure,

implying that the failing hospital site will continue to provide services post-merger. This will reduce the extent to which efficiency gains can be made and possibly result in a poor service being provided at the site which had faced insufficient demand. Of course, it may be possible to downsize rather than close the hospital, or to reorganise services between the two sites, in order to provide some minimum level at the site which has insufficient demand to support a full range of services.

However, in other cases the underlying demand might be sufficient to support a hospital but, owing to poor management or clinical performance, the quality of service is such that purchasers have withdrawn their business. Whilst this has indeed been cited as a driver for merger (Haggard, 1995), alternatives to rescuing such a Trust exist and merger might be a last resort rather than the best option.

6.5.7 Expansion of market power

The desire to increase market share and market power may also be a driver in some circumstances, especially for profit-making organisations. Whilst it is unlikely ever to be singled out as a driver for merger of Trusts in the UK (see Section 6.7), it has been studied in the USA, although even there hospitals are more likely to emphasise the potential efficiency gains from merger as they will be subject to antitrust challenges. Nevertheless, evidence to support this strategy in practice has been found. In a longitudinal study of three communities in the USA, Starkweather and Carman (1987) examined the nature of competition within and between hospital markets. In the area deemed to be most competitive, they explored the emergence of mergers between some of the seven hospitals, none of which originally had any degree of market power. Following a period of expansion and diversification by some of the hospitals in order to carve a market niche, they became aware of the futility of their individual competitive strategies and various proposals for merger arose.

By the end of the study period (five years), after several mergers and reconfigurations, the market was characterised as a differentiated oligopoly with a small number of dominant firms and a substantial part of the total market being produced by four corporations. The authors concluded that in this case study the strategy was certainly one of seeking to enhance market power: '. . . that of the numerous reasons advanced for mergers in industrial sectors and amongst hospitals in particular, a singular motivation was pursued in [this community]; in an era of increasing competition, the stronger hospitals moved with determination to reduce competition and establish domination. The fundamental motive was market control' (p194).

6.6 HOSPITAL MERGERS – GOOD OR BAD?

6.6.1 Availability and quality of evidence

It is clear from the theory that merger will have potential benefits and costs, hence policy in both the UK and the USA has been directed at assessing in advance the expected impact of merger proposals. However, what happens in practice once the merger has occurred is not well documented or understood. In the UK, no systematic evidence on post-merger performance or the impact of hospital mergers is collected and, as far as the authors are aware, no empirical work has been undertaken. Even in the USA where merger activity has been substantial and is seen by some to be the dominant strategy in the battle to capture shrinking healthcare dollars, commentators have noted the dearth of empirical evidence relating to the gains from hospital merger (Kassirer, 1996).

If the evidence from mergers in other sectors is used as a guide to what can be expected in the healthcare sector, then it would be concluded that many of the anticipated gains from mergers do not ever materialise. Comprehensive reviews of the literature in both the USA and the UK suggest that efficiency actually declines post-merger in many cases, owing to unforeseen problems in integration between the merging firms (Mueller, 1996).

It should be noted that there are significant methodological problems in interpreting results based on the post-merger performance of hospitals. Two specific problems are briefly referred to here; for a further discussion see Goddard and Ferguson (1997). The first relates to the nature of comparisons made, given the difficulty of attributing changes in certain variables to the merger event itself in a before-and-after approach. Some studies have attempted to reduce the degree of confounding by identifying a control group of non-merging hospitals with similar characteristics. Secondly, it is necessary to study merged hospitals for a long period of time following merger to capture all possible effects: this increases the likelihood of confounding through changes in the external environment which cannot easily be controlled for in any evaluation.

Notwithstanding these methodological issues, evidence is presented in the following section, based on direct comparisons either between pre- and post-merger hospitals or between merging and non-merging hospitals.

6.6.2 Direct evidence on hospital mergers

The author of one of the earliest studies examined 32 mergers of non-profit hospitals occurring between 1956 and 1970 (Treat, 1976). The dominant acquiring hospital was matched with a non-merging hospital and published data were used to create indicators of efficiency and effectiveness. Mean values for groups of merging and matched non-merging hospitals were calculated and their performance was compared in terms of the average change or mean difference in each indicator. Data were collected for the year before the merger and then for 3, 5 and 7 years post-merger to capture longer-term effects. The results indicated that the merging hospitals experienced a significant and ongoing increase in average cost per case, average cost per day and total expenditure.

Whilst the authors suggested that a short-term increase would be expected due to prospective costs (i.e. acquiring the organisation, updating facilities, etc.), the longer-term picture did not suggest that these were offset by any efficiency gains. Merging hospitals did not expand in terms of bed numbers as fast as their non-merging pairs, although reductions in bed numbers were rare. In terms of effectiveness indicators, the merging hospitals produced a greater range of services than their counterparts. The evidence on all other variables was inconclusive.

The most important aspect of this analysis is revealed by sub-analysis of hospitals based on their size and whether they are located in a rural or urban area. Small hospitals (under 300 beds) and hospitals in more rural areas performed well on the indicator of labour intensity which suggested that they had been able to attract more personnel. The authors interpreted this as a positive sign, given that small and rural hospitals often found it hard to recruit and hold qualified personnel. Additionally, rural hospitals (all of which had fewer than 300 beds) were the only ones which achieved a reduced average cost per case, reduced length of stay and higher occupancy rates over time than the non-merging counterparts. Thus the authors conclude that mergers appear to be very viable for small rural facilities but that the benefits for larger, urban hospitals are more questionable and cast doubt on the economies of scale argument for merger.

During the 1980s, the healthcare environment changed substantially and it might be expected that mergers occurring in later years would have a different impact. Several studies have looked at mergers which occurred during this period. Mullner and Andersen (1987) examined the impact of mergers during the period 1980–85, distinguishing between acquired hospitals (55), acquiring hospitals (45) and those which consolidated by forming a new entity (62 hospitals forming 32 new entities in total). Data were collected from published sources for each merging hospital for the year prior to merger and for each consolidated entity for one year before and one year after the consolidation. These were compared with data for all other hospitals in the USA at the mid-point of the study. Measures of institutional characteristics included size, type of service, ownership and occupancy rate.

Most mergers involved a larger hospital acquiring a smaller one and most of the acquiring hospitals had above-average occupancy rates. Location characteristics included metropolitan versus non-metropolitan area and size of the community in which the merger occurred. A large proportion of merged and consolidated hospitals were in metropolitan areas, which typically had larger communities. Financial characteristics included measures of short-term liquidity and overall profitability which were calculated for the five years preceding merger and up to four years afterwards, standardised to control for changes in the hospital industry over time. These indicated that hospitals involved in either merger or consolidation were financially close to the industry averages and that no clear financial gains or losses characterised those hospitals either before or after merger (or consolidation). However, the use of financial ratios has been criticised on the grounds that these may hide offsetting financial effects which leave the ratio unchanged (Woodward, 1987).

Greene (1990) reports on a survey of 36 hospitals which merged into 18 institutions between 1985 and 1987. Data on operating and financial characteristics were analysed for two years prior to merger, the merger year and two years following merger. The revenue and expenditure figures were adjusted for geographical variations in labour costs and revenues, and expenditure figures were standardised to control for case-mix differences, but no attempt was made to provide data on industry averages or matched comparisons in order to control for changes in the external environment. One interesting feature of this survey was the distinction between costs and charges which can indicate whether any efficiency savings achieved by merger actually reduce costs to purchasers, or are retained by the merged hospital in the form of higher profits. Immediately following the merger, most financial indicators illustrated a down-turn, which was attributed to, for instance, problems of aligning cultures and poor staff morale.

Financial prospects improved one and two years following the merger, but, although expenditure was reduced, the study found that charges were increased, which contributed to increased profitability by around 4 per cent over two years. The author concludes that these findings appear to contradict the hospital industry's claim that mergers can help to reduce healthcare costs to consumers. The survey responses suggest that merger proposals should place less emphasis on financial benefits to the community, especially in the short-term, and more on quality and innovation. Large financial benefits appear to be achievable only if one facility closes or is converted to a non-acute use, but due to the unpopularity of such proposals amongst staff and the public, these options are rarely stated in merger plans.

The short-term effects of 92 hospital mergers which took place between 1982–89 were examined in a study which controlled for secular trends by using a random group of non-merging hospitals for comparative purposes (Alexander et al, 1996). Published data were used to consider the impact of merger on three areas of operation:

- scale of activity (measured by numbers of staffed beds and admissions);
- staffing practices (measured by total number of personnel and number of nurses);
- operating efficiency (measured by occupancy rates and total expenditure per admission).

Data from the three years before and after merger were used to calculate mean values and rates of change for each variable. Mergers were stratified by three categories: size similarity, ownership similarity and period of merger. It could be expected that changes in operational variables would be more evident where: (1) merging hospitals are of dissimilar size (as the dominant hospital would be able to force changes on the smaller one); (2) ownership is similar (as common ownership status may reflect similar values and orientation which facilitate change); and (3) mergers occur more recently (as they face greater financial pressures from PPS).

The results show that the greatest impact is on operating efficiency rather than on the other variables. Although occupancy rates fell after merger, the rate of change was significantly lower in the merging hospitals than elsewhere. Similarly, increases in expenditure per admission were seen after merger but these were lower than the increase in non-merging hospitals. It is suggested that the merged hospitals were able to improve operating efficiency relative to non-merging hospitals by slowing the trends towards higher costs and lower occupancy rates that were occurring in the industry as a whole. This improvement was not, however, apparent in terms of before-and-after comparisons of the merging hospitals.

A more technical approach to the evaluation of efficiency gains or losses from merger considered 79 mergers occurring between 1980 and 1988 in the USA, attempting to measure productive and scale efficiencies using data envelopment analysis (Fried and Yaisawarng, 1994). For each merger case, aggregate pre-merger and post-merger efficiency indices were created and compared, where the pre-merger index represented the predicted efficiency of the merged unit if merger had no effect on efficiency. The study used three types of returns to scale scenarios and various specifications of input and output. Using published data, the authors concluded that of the 53 mergers on which they had sufficient post-merger data, 39 of them experienced an average post-merger gain in productive efficiency of 9.8 per cent; 12 experienced an average loss of 9.4 per cent and two neither gained nor lost. This suggests a 5 per cent net efficiency gain from mergers compared to their predicted efficiency had they not merged.

Investigation of the outcome of hospital mergers in the context of multihospital systems has been undertaken by Dranove and Shanley (1996). They confine their analysis to systems which are defined as two or more physically separate hospitals sharing common ownership. Their study considers the characteristics of 13 local hospital systems and compares them with non-system hospitals. A Monte Carlo approach is taken to choose the latter group, ensuring that they contain the same number of hospitals and comparable numbers of beds to those in the systems. The hypothesis being tested is that system hospitals may be able to reduce costs and achieve reputation benefits through the exploitation of economies of scale and scope. The authors conclude that whilst their analysis provides some support for the existence of reputation benefits linked to marketing strategies, it does not support the view that significant cost reductions accrue from hospital merger through the exploitation of other economies of scale such as administrative or production economies. The authors also summarise previous empirical research on hospital chains and conclude that this has produced mixed results.

6.6.3 Summary of direct evidence

The research highlights the distinction between location and ownership which needs to be considered in determining the impact of mergers. Hospital chains are becoming more common in the USA but are less relevant to the UK healthcare sector at present as the ownership (or, more accurately, the management) of NHS Trusts is limited to the hospitals within a local area and a single Trust. Thus spatial monopoly is the focus within the NHS. However, where hospital chains are local, the findings are more relevant as they at least suggest that there may be potential benefits from consolidating physical plant.

Overall however, the results from these studies are clearly inconclusive. Those which attempt to control for confounding variables are likely to be the most methodologically sound and their results can be given more weight. The results remain unconvincing, suggesting that the predicted efficiency gains of merger do not always appear and that unexpected costs often arise. Although additional costs can be expected in the shorter term, especially where new capital developments are undertaken as part of the process, the unexpected costs are usually associated with difficulties in integrating systems and personnel from two different organisations. For example, some case studies have noted the need to make adjustments both to incompatible information systems and to salaries in order to maintain parity (Anderson, 1991). Most studies have focused on financial variables and changes in the range of services offered, owing to the difficulties associated with measuring other vari-

ables such as quality of services, especially over relatively short time periods.

6.7 REGIONAL OFFICE SURVEY

It is not straightforward to examine how UK policy has been applied to the NHS, since much of the data and evidence used in the assessment and decision-making processes do not appear in the public domain. This is particularly true where the merger is below whole-Trust level, or does not require the dissolution of a Trust, since no ministerial approval is needed in such cases. Furthermore, it is not clear how far Regional Offices (which are responsible for implementing most of the processes involved) would be held to account for failing to ensure that the national guidance is followed.

To shed some light on this, a questionnaire was sent to all of the eight UK Regional Offices which could be expected to act as the 'local regulators' in considering merger proposals. Three Regions (38 per cent) completed the short questionnaire which attempted to elicit, for specific mergers which had taken place in the Region concerned, the main factors driving mergers. Those completing the questionnaire were asked to identify the three main drivers for each merger, and to prioritise these. In the second part of the questionnaire, respondents were asked to explain how the national guidance had been used in the assessment process, and to identify which parts of the process were considered most/least useful.

In total, eight mergers were involved across the three Regions for which questionnaires were completed. None of these cases involved mergers below Trust level. Clearly it is impossible to identify a robust pattern of responses from such a small sample. Nevertheless, there is evidence to support the view that concentrating services to: (1) meet medical training/accreditation requirements, (2) meet national policy guidance on service delivery and (3) improve service quality, are consistently important factors behind mergers. One of these factors was seen as the most important driver in seven of the eight mergers considered. In the remaining case, insufficient demand to support more than one hospital was cited as the main reason for merger.

Interestingly, purchasers were viewed as initiating the impetus for merger in approximately half the cases. Where this was the case, integration of care and cost savings were typically quoted, with possible loss of competition or choice seen as the main drawbacks. In general, respondents considered that if benefits were to be realised, this would only be in the longer-term. Reference was made to the lack of post-project evaluation and clear criteria upon which to measure benefits.

In terms of how merger policy is applied, the responses indicate a certain scepticism that an all-encompassing national policy can be defined. Reference was made to the need to take into account local circumstances, supplementing the guidance criteria with other factors. Perhaps the most important point here is to ensure that national policy can be applied flexibly, adopting a case-by-case approach. It is not, however, an argument against having a more explicit framework within which to define and measure the costs and benefits of merger.

An interesting point made by one respondent related to *how* the merger process would actually take place once the decision had been taken to merge. Merger should, it was argued, be viewed as an output (for which there exist alternatives, such as takeover or dissolution) and the focus should be upon how the actual reconfiguration of services should take place. This to some extent echoes the recommendation in the relevant Effective Health Care Bulletin (Volume 2, Number 8, 1996) that the onus should lie with those proposing merger to demonstrate precisely *how* cost savings or benefits will be realised.

6.8 CONCLUSION

The evidence on the impact of mergers in the healthcare sector is inconclusive. Where evidence from the literature is available, it suggests that the expected benefits from merger are frequently not realised. Unexpected costs which have been reported in the literature include difficulties associated with integrating systems and personnel from the merging organisations.

There are many reasons proposed for hospital mergers and it is important to disentangle

these when assessing the costs and benefits prospectively. Mergers which are proposed as a means of reducing excess capacity could be expected to have a greater impact on cost structures than where two existing organisations are operating 'efficiently' but still planning to merge services. Most studies have focused upon financial variables and changes in the range of services offered, owing to difficulties in measuring more qualitative features of service. Potentially this is important given the emphasis placed upon improved quality of service as a key benefit of mergers. For example, many service reviews conclude that different services should be concentrated on a single site to maximise the benefits from links between specialties (technically referred to as economies of scope with respect to quality).

The results from our limited Regional Office survey confirm the importance attached to improvements in service quality as a perceived benefit of merger. They also point, however, to other important drivers such as medical training/accreditation requirements. Such factors ought to be accorded sufficient attention in a framework for assessing the advantages and disadvantages of merger. Financial considerations, although clearly important, may be given a disproportionate weight simply because they are – at least superficially – easier to measure.

No formal, systematic evaluation has been undertaken of mergers in the NHS, either prospectively or retrospectively. It is recognised in Department of Health guidance that mergers can take place at the level of whole hospital Trusts or with regard to specific services. Evaluation of the latter is particularly important given the likelihood that political factors will tend to favour solutions which avoid the closure of whole hospital sites (assuming that in at least some cases this will be a consequence of merger proposals). Whether dealing with whole-hospital or service mergers, it is critical that a more explicit framework for evaluation is used to assess the costs and benefits of merger proposals. Reports that hospital mergers may be viewed as a way of achieving significant healthcare cost savings are particularly worrying in view of evidence which clearly shows that the case for merger remains 'not proven'.

REFERENCES

Alexander J A, Halpern M T, Lee S D 1996 The Short-Term Effects of Merger on Hospital Operations. Health Services Research 30:827–847.

Anderson H J 1991 Hospitals Face Tough Issues in Years Following Mergers. Hospitals 65:24–32.

British Paediatric Association (BPA) 1993 The Care of Critically Ill Children. Report of a Multidisciplinary Working Party on Intensive Care, BPA London.

Calman K 1993 Hospital Doctors: Training for the Future. Department of Health, London.

Craig N, Forbes J 1996 Blind Choice or Informed Faith? Cognitive Dissonance and Competition in Health Care. Paper to HESG, January 1996.

Dawson D 1995 Regulating Competition in the NHS: The Department of Health Guide on Mergers and Anti-Competitive Behaviour. University of York Discussion Paper 131, York.

Department of Health 1993 Making London Better. HMSO, London.

Department of Health 1995 A Policy Framework for Commissioning Cancer Services. A report by the Expert Advisory Group on Cancer Services to the Chief Medical Officers of England and Wales. HMSO, London.

Department of Justice and Federal Trade Commission (DOJ/FTC) 1992 Statement Accompanying Release of Revised Merger Guidelines. April 2 1992, Washington.

Dranove D, Durkac A, Shanley M 1996 Are Multihospital Systems More Efficient? Health Affairs 15:100–104.

Effective Health Care Bulletin 1996 Hospital Volume and Health Care Outcomes, Costs and Patient Access. 2:8.

Ferguson B, Posnett J 1994 Pricing in the NHS Internal Market. Health Economics 3: 133–136.

Fried HO, Yaisawarng S 1994 Hospital Mergers and Efficiency. Seminar Paper No. 12/95 – Monash University.

Goddard M, Ferguson B 1997 'Mergers in the NHS: Made in Heaven or Marriages of Convenience?' Nuffield Provincial Hospital Trust Occasional Paper (forthcoming).

Greene J 1990 Do Mergers Work? Modern Healthcare 19: 24–33.

Greene J 1992 The Costs of Hospital Mergers. Modern Healthcare 3: 36–43.

Haggard L 1995 Smooth Moves. In Managing Mergers, Health Services Journal. Macmillan, London.

Harrison A, Prentice S 1996 Acute Futures. King's Fund, London.

Health and Personal Social Services Statistics 1996 HMSO, London.

Health Services Journal 1994 Trusts will Break Law in Tendering for Hospital Sites. 4 August: 7.

Health Services Journal 1995 Merger no Solution to New Deal. 3 August: 6.

Health Services Journal 1996 Welsh Hospitals faced with Closure or Radical Change. 11 July: 5.

Health Services Journal 1996 In Brief – Pembrokeshire and Derwen Trust Interested in Merger. 18 July: 6.

Health Services Journal 1996 Trust Merger Mooted to End Funding and Staff. 18 July: 9.

Health Services Journal 1996 HA Aims to Cut County's Seven Trusts to Three. 15 August: 5.

Health Services Journal 1996 Trust Chiefs Clash over Merger Plan. 31 October: 8.

Health Services Journal 1997 Birmingham Hospitals in Merger Ruckus. 23 January: 4.

The Independent 1997 Labour's £2 billion plan to shut down hospitals. 24 March 1997.

Jarman B 1993 Is London Overbedded? British Medical Journal 306:979–982.

Kassirer J P 1996 Mergers and Acquisitions – Who Benefits? Who Loses? The New England Journal of Medicine 334: 722–723.

Lazarus A 1995 The Effect of Mergers and Acquisitions on Behavioural Health Care. Medical Interface 8:103–106.

Leeds Review Task Force 1996 The Leeds Review of Acute Hospital Services. Final Report, Leeds Review Task Force, Leeds.

Miller R H 1996 Competition in the Health System: Good News and Bad News. Health Affairs 15: 107–120.

Mueller D C 1996 Lessons from the United State's Antitrust History. International Journal of Industrial Organisation 14:415–445.

Mullner R M, Andersen RM 1987 A Descriptive and Financial Ratio Analysis of Merged and Consolidated Hospitals: United States 1980–1985. Advances in Health Economics and Health Services Research 7: 41–58.

NAHAT 1994 The Future of Provider Services: Trusts Mergers and De-Mergers.

NHS Centre for Reviews and Dissemination 1995 Which Way Forward for the Care of Critically Ill Children? CRD Report 1, University of York.

NHS Executive 1994 The Operation of the NHS Internal Market: Local Freedoms, National Responsibilities. HMSO, London.

Oxfordshire Health Authority 1996 The Number of NHS Trusts in Oxfordshire. A Report to the Authority paper 96/68, December 1996.

Redmayne S 1995 Reshaping the NHS, Strategies, Priorities and Resource Allocation. NAHAT, Birmingham.

Redmayne S 1996 Small Steps, Big Goals: Purchasing Policies in the NHS. NAHAT, Birmingham.

Robinson J, Casalino L 1996 Vertical Integration and Organisational Networks in Health Care. Health Affairs, Spring: 7–21.

Starkweather D B, Carman J M 1987 Horizontal and Vertical Concentrations in the Evolution of Hospital Competition. Advances in Health Economics and Health Services Research 7: 179–194.

Tomlinson B 1992 Report of the Inquiry into London's Health Service, Medical Education and Research. HMSO, London.

Treat T F 1976 The Performance of Merging Hospitals. Medical Care 14:199–209.

Turner J 1994 Current Issues in Acute Care: Re-configuring Acute Services I. IHSM, London.

Turner J 1995 Current Issues in Acute Care: Re-configuring Acute Services II. IHSM, London.

Turner J 1996 Current Issues in Acute Care: Re-configuring Acute Services III. IHSM, London.

Vickers J, Hay D 1987 The Economics of Market Dominance. In The Economics of Market Dominance (eds) Hay D, Vickers J, Blackwell, Oxford 1987.

Vistnes G 1995 Hospital Mergers and Antitrust Enforcement. Journal of Health Politics, Policy and Law 20:175–190.

Vita M G, Langenfield J, Pautler P, Miller L 1991 Economic Analysis in Health Care Antitrust. Journal of Contemporary Health Law and Policy 7:73–115.

Woodward A 1987 Comments on Ratio Analysis of Merged Hospitals. Advances in Health Economics and Health Services Research 7:115–117.

7

Impact on the purchaser–provider relationship and implications for the regulatory framework

Maria Goddard, Brian Ferguson, John Posnett

7.1 INTRODUCTION

Preceding chapters have examined the evidence relating to the impact of concentration of hospital services on costs, quality and access and have explored some of the factors which are currently driving concentration. The purpose of this chapter is to consider the role of regulation in addressing some of the issues raised by further service concentration in the NHS, and to assess the appropriateness of the current regulatory framework. Suggestions are also made regarding the future direction of policy.

7.2 THE ECONOMIC BASIS FOR REGULATION

Before reviewing the issues and policies relating to concentration in the specific context of the NHS, it is worth examing briefly the development of general Competition Law and regulatory policy in other sectors, especially in the privatised utilities, which share some of the characteristics of the NHS market. This will illustrate the economic basis for regulation as well as providing some useful parallels with the NHS regulatory framework.

The development of general Competition Law in the UK is predicated on the implicit assumption that market power is undesirable, allowing firms to drive up prices in order to make 'excess' profits and to create welfare losses. Thus the policy emphasis has been on restricting routes to the acquisition of market power and dealing with the potential abuse of market power if it arises (Williams, 1993). Much of current policy reflects the structure–conduct–performance (SCP) paradigm, based on neo-classical economic theory, which was popular in the 1950s and 1960s (e.g. Bain, 1956). This holds that there is a causal relationship between the market structure in which firms operate and their conduct and subsequent economic performance. Structure is determined by a variety of factors, including the number and size of buyers and sellers in the market, the extent to which products in that market are differentiated and the ease of entry by new firms. These factors influence the conduct of firms within the market, including the method of price setting, investment strategy, and expenditure on research and innovation; these together determine performance in terms of economic efficiency and consumer welfare.

Much of the empirical work undertaken by economists has focused on one particular element of structure – the level of market concentration (see Ferguson and Ferguson, 1994, for a review). Grounded in neo-classical theory and emphasising the welfare properties of a perfectly competitive market, the SCP paradigm suggests that markets characterised by many buyers and sellers with small market shares (low concentration), low entry barriers and a homogeneous product are likely to perform better as allocative and technical efficiency will be maximised, no excess profits will be made and consumer welfare will be maximised. In contrast, markets involving few sellers with large market shares (high concentration) are likely to perform poorly owing to the existence of market power. In particular, firms in highly concentrated markets have the ability to make excess profits and a large body of empirical research has supported the existence of a link between concentration and high levels of profit in various industries (Norman and La Manna, 1992).

One implication of this approach is that regulatory policy should be aimed at retaining a competitive structure where possible and dealing with anti-competitive behaviour where it arises. The limitations of focusing solely on market concentration as a measure of structure was highlighted in the theory of contestable markets (Baumol et al, 1982) and subsequently influenced the development of competition policy. The ability of a single firm or group of firms to exploit market power depends on factors other than current market concentration, one crucial factor being the extent to which barriers to entry prevent the entry of new firms attracted by high profits, which will ensure a return to more competitive levels. The abuse of market power can be offset even in a highly concentrated market if entry is unrestricted, because actual entry or threat of entry by new firms makes the market contestable, thereby forcing the incumbent firms to behave *as if they were in a competitive environment.*[1]

General competition policy has therefore been aimed at blocking potential routes to market power, which include collusion with competitors, merger with competitors, and anti-competitive practices to deter entry, or to force the exit of competitors from the market. The Restrictive Trade Practices Act (RTPA) and the Resale Prices Act (RPA) are aimed at preventing collusive behaviour; policy derived from the Fair Trading Act (FTA) deals with mergers; and the FTA and Competition Act (CA) deal with anti-competitive practices (Williams, 1993). As competition policy may not be successful in preventing the acquisition of market power, the FTA allows the potential abuse of market power to be investigated and dealt with, where necessary, by the Monopolies and Mergers Commission (MMC). This approach suggests that the need for regulation will be greater where the possibility of market power is greatest and this is reflected in the development of industry-specific regulatory policy in the privatised utilities.

Before outlining the regulatory policy in the privatised utilities and drawing some parallels with the NHS situation, it is important to note that this approach to monopoly and hence to regulation is not without detractors. The validity of the SCP approach was called into question in the 1970s by economists (the 'Chicago School') who emphasised the dynamic properties of the market and argued that the observed statistical relationship between the level of concentration and profitability of firms did not necessarily represent a *causal* link. They interpreted the existence of high profits in some markets as a sign of efficiency rather than market power, arguing that, over time, those firms with the lowest costs will tend to increase in size and obtain higher market shares and profits as a result of their superior efficiency (Demsetz, 1973). At the same time, alternative theoretical perspectives moved away from the emphasis on structure to focus more closely on the conduct of firms and their strategic behaviour. Firms were viewed not as reacting solely to their environment but as making strategic decisions which take into account the reactions of others in the market and the subsequent impact on their environment (Norman and La Manna, 1992; Jacquemin, 1987).

This type of analysis allows for the introduction of a large set [2] of possible outcomes from co-operative and non-co-operative behaviour amongst firms (e.g. see Slade and Jacquemin, 1992), but still operates within the neo-classical framework. The 'Austrian School' of economists departed from the traditional neo-classical theory in a number of ways, [3] but the key element in relation to the analysis of markets and market power is the focus on the dynamic processes of markets and the role of entrepreneurial activity. The latter can produce welfare gains through innovation and technical progress, whereby the existence of high profits in some markets may reflect the rewards for innovation, skill and foresight. Also, market power is in any case likely to be transitory (e.g. Kirzner, 1973). In addition, the 'New Institutional Economics' emphasises the circumstances in which particular organisational structures and relationships between market players, which may appear to be anti-competitive when judged in terms of traditional theory and the SCP approach, may actually be more efficient (Williamson, 1985, 1989).

Clearly, these theoretical developments tend to view issues related to market power in a very different way. Although many of these developments have had some influence on the way in which competition policy has evolved, [4] the SCP paradigm and neo-classical theory have had the largest influence on policy development in the UK and the USA (for a review of the latter, see Mueller, 1996). As Williams (1993) notes, whilst the Austrian and Chicago schools may favour free markets, which are thought to produce the best outcomes even at the expense of high levels of concentration and apparent market power, the underlying premise of competition policy is that competition should be encouraged but that the free market may not be compatible with the maintenance of competition. This suggests a role for some form of Government intervention.

7.3 REGULATION OF PRIVATISED UTILITIES

In addition to the four statutes which comprise general Competition Law (RTPA, RPA, FTA, CA), a body of industry-specific regulation has arisen as national industries have been privatised. Starting with the privatisation of British Telecom in 1984, regulatory bodies have been set up for each of the utilities, each formally independent of Government and headed by a Director General. Superficially, the introduction of regulatory frameworks for the privatised utilities appeared contradictory: on the one hand, the rationale for privatisation was the belief that the industries were inefficient, partly as a result of being protected from the discipline of competition and being subjected to interference from ministers within a confusing and contradictory system of rules and regulations (Veljanovski, 1991); on the other hand, the regulatory bodies were set up with various powers which restricted the behaviour of the newly privatised companies, and which could be seen as stifling the very behaviour which the Government wished to encourage in its privatisation programme. The economic rationale for such apparently contradictory behaviour relates to the nature of the markets within which the utilities operated.[5] If competition is expected to flourish, preventing the acquisition and exercise of market power, there is no need for regulation; however, if the market exhibits 'failures' which suggest that, left to itself, it will not produce the desired outcomes, a potential role for regulation exists. Whilst it is not necessary to go into detail here, the major failure for most of the utilities is the existence of a natural monopoly,[6] which raises issues of market power. [7]

Much of the economic regulatory activity that the regulators of the privatised utilities undertake is concerned with the consequences of natural monopoly. In most of these industries there is a combination of activities, some of which are naturally monopolistic, such as transmission networks, (e.g. electricity grids, local telecommunications lines, gas pipelines, sewerage networks, rail track and stations); whilst others are potentially competitive, such as the supply of services which require access to the former activities (e.g. long-distance calls, generation and supply of gas and electricity, train services). Although some elements of production or service provision may be *potentially* competitive, the regulators have needed to ensure that this potential has been realised in a number of cases. For example, British Gas was transferred to the private sector as a fully integrated monopoly (which has led some commentators (Stelzer, 1991) to observe that the British, in contrast to the USA, have an 'aversion' to competition) and it has taken a long time for structural regulation to have an impact on competition in supply. In contrast, the privatisation of the electricity industry was accompanied by regulation to break up both vertical and horizontal constraints in generation and transmission activities, as well as a regional structure for distribution and retail supply (Armstrong et al, 1995). Recent developments in the rail industry have focused on both regional and vertical separation.

7.4 REGULATORY POLICY IN THE NHS[8]

7.4.1 Importance of structure on the supply side

A central theme of the NHS reforms was the introduction of competition on the supply side of the internal market. However, there is clearly a strong locational element in the provision of many types of healthcare services, which when coupled with the widely held belief in the potential for economies of scale and scope [9] (Le Grand and Bartlett, 1993), suggests that concentration of services is likely to

arise. As illustrated in the previous chapter, merger activity at the level of the hospital, specialty and service has been substantial and there are no signs that this is abating. In recognition of this, and in order to reiterate the importance of supply-side competition and contestability, the Department of Health outlined its regulatory policy in the 1994 guidance, 'The Operation of the NHS Internal Market: Local Freedoms, National Responsibilities' (NHS Executive, 1994). The guidance noted that, 'competition provides the stimulus for ... services to be efficient and to respond to the needs of patients and the public' and that, '... [purchasers] need to have a choice of providers to get the best possible service. For many services it is therefore efficient to have competition between several providers. For other services ... it may be more efficient to have just one provider, whose behaviour is stimulated by the knowledge that another provider could replace it' (p3). If monopoly is the most efficient way of organising the production of some services, the need to regulate conduct is also acknowledged.

7.4.2 Provider mergers

Concentration is addressed in the policy on provider mergers between whole NHS Trusts and also mergers at the service or specialty level. The stated goal of the policy is to allow mergers or joint ventures with net beneficial effects to go ahead, but to ensure that 'proposed mergers/joint ventures do not lead to the acquisition and abuse of monopoly power, with subsequent detrimental effects on patient welfare' (p10). A local decision limit, defined by market share (for mergers) and size (for joint ventures) is set out with the aim of allowing mergers which fall into this category to proceed without investigation as they are unlikely to have a significant effect on competition. Policy-specific clauses are added to exclude particular activities from the decision limit (e.g. all mergers between acute and community Trusts) and an 'exceptional circumstances' clause is also included.

The guidance outlines the nature of the assessment process for merger activity which falls outside the limits and is therefore investigated. The aim is to quantify the impact on competition and, in cases where this is likely to have a negative effect, to assess whether any compensating economic or non-economic factors are sufficient to produce overall net benefits. The steps in the assessment of merger proposals are as follows:

(1) **Measuring the Impact on Competition:**

- defining the service and the market;
- measuring the extent of concentration in that market;
- assessing the probability of entry by other suppliers.

(2) **Estimation of other Benefits:**

- economic benefits;
- non-economic benefits.

Step 1 involves the definition of the economic market, based on travelling time zones around each provider (p17). For A&E services, a 14 or 19 minute travel time zone (urban and rural areas respectively) is used, based on Patients' Charter standards for ambulance response times; for other services, the zone is set at 30 minutes. Concentration is defined in terms of the number of providers and the proportion of activity accounted for in a given geographical area: in other words, on the basis of market share, but with no subsequent calculation of concentration indices.[10] Cut-off points are used to define areas of low, medium and high concentration and these are intended to be a function of the maximum travel times recommended for certain services such as A&E.

The *probability of entry* is included in the assessment because if entry is likely to occur in a timely way in response to the exercise of monopoly power, then the market is contestable even if it is dominated by one or few providers. Factors to be considered in making an assessment on entry are listed: for example, the possibility of other Trusts having spare capacity, and entry from the private and voluntary sectors.

Step 2 considers the *potential benefits* from merger which may offset any loss of competition. The economic benefits relate to the efficiency arguments for merger and are listed as economies of scale and scope in relation to both costs and quality of service. Examples of situations in which efficiency may be enhanced are listed and an Appendix summarises the published literature relating to economies of scale and scope, although it recommends that it would be '... unwise to base decisions on the organisation of hospital services on the basis of this literature alone' (p23). The non-economic benefits include the creation of employment opportunities and the implications of closure of new units with recent investment or of units popular with the public (this assumes that merger is acting to prevent failure in some circumstances).

The responsibilities of various parties are listed, with the Regional Offices taking the main role in assessment and decision-making, and the burden of proof for the benefits of merger resting with the merging parties.

7.4.3 Providers in difficulty – managing exit

One of the key incentives provided by a competitive environment is that suppliers who provide the quality of services required by consumers at an acceptable price are rewarded by winning business, whereas those who perform badly face losses and ultimately exit from the market. In addition to providing incentives to firms within the market, exit is clearly linked with the structure of the market as (along with entry) it determines the number and type of firms.

In the NHS, providers do in principle face this discipline as dissatisfied purchasers can shift contracts elsewhere. As expenditure is largely cash-limited, 'winning' providers are rewarded at the expense of 'losers' which face reduced activity levels. In practice, the purchasing process is complex and there are many reasons why this mechanism may not work adequately,[11] with providers often unlikely to find themselves exposed to the discipline of competitive forces. Instead, a range of other options have emerged for dealing with poor performance, including the financial 'bailing out' of poorly performing Trusts through the use of Health Authority or Regional Office transitional funding (as a loan or gift), or merger with a stronger Trust. These actions may give poor incentives for Trusts to perform well and may encourage Trusts to adopt strategies without due regard to the risk involved, as they may expect to be rescued if the strategy fails. Opting for merger rather than exit may be appropriate in some circumstances, but the danger of failing to analyse carefully the cause of the poor performance is that merger may be chosen for the wrong reason. For example, if poor management or clinical quality is central to the problem, it may be preferable to allow 'exit' of the management or clinical team, thereby avoiding significant changes in the structure of the market brought about by orchestrating 'arranged marriages' to deal with the problem. A case has arisen where a Trust appears likely to exit the NHS due to lack of purchaser support (Health Services Journal, 26 September 1996), but there are many more instances where Trusts have been in difficulty but less explicit solutions have been found.

The regulatory guidance seeks to remedy this situation by setting out an explicit process, firstly for deciding whether a Trust really is in financial difficulty or is just facing a transient, soluble problem; and secondly, if the Trust *is* in difficulty, providing a set of options for deciding what action should be taken. The key to deciding what action should be taken when Trusts are in difficulty is to pinpoint the *cause* of the problem, as poor performance or inefficiency will not always be the cause. The existence of excess capacity in the acute sector was highlighted by the NHS reforms, especially in urban areas where several Trusts offered similar services in a relatively small area. Much of this has been addressed through the 'managed' exit of services and providers (e.g. Tomlinson, 1992; Department of Health, 1993). Continued pressure on purchasers' budgets and the shift to a primary care-led NHS implies that lack of resources and spare capacity are likely to persist and will be dealt with through various forms of reconfiguration. In such cases, exit is not necessarily related directly to the effects of competition.

The guidance seeks to distinguish between short-term deficits and indications of longer term non-viability by listing a set of criteria by which the Regional Office can assess financial viability. A 'local decision limit' within which the NHS Executive will not take any action is set to allow Trusts facing specific financial problems to deal with them independently if the problems are relatively small, or if they are larger but have been foreseen and can be remedied with a specific plan. Allowance is made for the fact that poor management of a Trust may be one reason why the Trust is failing, but that under a different management it may be viable in the long run (p39).

Proposals to sharpen incentives by distinguishing more carefully between 'real' reasons for failing to meet financial duties and 'technical' reasons (due to accounting and pricing rules) have recently been put forward, aimed at making the achievement of financial duties a better indicator of financial performance (NHS Executive, 1996).

7.4.4 Regulation of conduct

The Department of Health's approach mirrors that taken by the regulators of privatised utilities by placing limits on the conduct of organisations which hold market power. There are two main elements to the Department of Health's policy on conduct: pricing policy which impinges on NHS Trusts, and policy directed at collusive behaviour, which concerns both Trusts and purchasers. Pricing issues are not discussed in the regulatory guidance but constitute one element of the financial regime faced by NHS Trusts since the start of the reforms.

7.4.5 Pricing and costing policy

Trusts are required to set the prices they charge to NHS purchasers equal to the average total cost of providing each service. Cross-subsidisation between contracts is not allowed and marginal cost pricing is allowed only for the sale of unplanned excess capacity. Other financial duties of Trusts have a bearing on the pricing regime: they are required to break even, taking one year with another; achieve a 6 per cent return on the average value of net assets; and meet their external financing limit (EFL).[12] At present, Trusts have little incentive to improve efficiency as any planned surplus made through reducing costs will affect the following year's EFL. Although Trusts are allowed to retain unplanned savings in the year they are generated, the following year they are required to reduce prices to reflect the lower costs. Whilst this might in principle attract more business from purchasers, the Trust does not benefit directly from the reduced costs as the savings are (at least in theory) passed on to the purchaser. This is in contrast to the regulated utilities where providers are free to retain gains for (in theory) five years. The drawbacks of the NHS approach have been documented by Propper (1995).

The costing and pricing rules were devised at the outset of the reforms to ensure a degree of openness in information between providers and purchasers, and to prevent providers from treating purchasers differently, depending in part on the degree of market power they had (NHS Executive, 1996). The apparent discrepancy between the accounting procedures used to allocate costs (especially the costs of jointly used assets) led the Department of Health to issue rules setting out the standard costing procedures to be used (NHS Management Executive, 1993).

However, in recognition of the fact that the current system offers some disincentives for efficient and innovative behaviour, there have recently been proposals for liberalisation of the pricing regime (NHS Executive, 1996). In particular, a survey of Trusts revealed that although there were many perceived benefits from the current system, relaxation of the cost = price rule might bring other benefits, including:

- a better reward system with incentives for good management;
- flexibility for funding future service developments;
- an incentive for developing better costing mechanisms (KPMG, 1996).

It is not possible to give full details of the proposals here, but they reflect an approach aimed at balancing innovative and responsive behaviour with the prevention of monopoly power abuse in particular services and locations. To this end, although the proposals recommend the ultimate removal of the cost = price rule to allow Trusts to price most services according to market conditions and to earn and spend surpluses in excess of 6 per cent, this can only happen following an increase in transparency, such as the publication of comparative prices for a common set of procedures, a sharper exit regime and a more sophisticated approach to costing.

7.4.6 Collusive behaviour

The second main regulatory tool used to combat the abuse of market power is the guidance on collusive behaviour. This covers collusion between providers and between purchasers and providers, the latter reflecting the not unusual situation of bilateral monopoly. The policy is aimed at establishing in particular cases whether collusion is inefficient, limiting its effects (largely through encouraging competition) and taking action where it is identified. A distinction is made between *co-operation,* which is in the interests of patients (including the sharing of large investments between providers, joint negotiation of contracts, longer-term contracts between purchasers and providers) and *collusion,* which is in the interests of providers (and sometimes purchasers) and which may lead to the acquisition and abuse of market power.

Examples of collusive behaviour are given: price-fixing, market-sharing agreements, collusive provider tendering for contracts, lack of competition at the contract renewal stage, and unjustifiable purchaser support for inefficient units. The difficulties of detection are acknowledged, especially as providers may engage in tacit rather than overt collusion (p48). The penalties for collusion are cancellation of the collusive contracts and 'management action' (p50).

7.5 ASSESSMENT OF POLICY

Setting aside the issues about whether or not competition is desirable in healthcare and also the debate about whether the market should be left to its own devices or regulated in order to promote competition, the question here is the extent to which the current regulatory policy is likely to achieve its *stated* aims.

7.5.1 Discretionary nature of policy

One of the features of effective regulatory policy is that it should enhance certainty for those in the market by making clear the conditions under which regulation applies and by making the decision-making process more transparent. This is acknowledged in NHS policy: 'where NHS Executive intervention is needed it will have clear aims and be on the basis of explicit criteria, so that participants know where they stand and so far as possible can predict the outcome' (p5). However, some of the features of the current regime appear to militate against this and involve instead a great deal of interpretation and discretion.

There are several areas in which the guidance is vague and leaves open the type of information required or the way in which information will be interpreted. An example arises in the assessment process for merger proposals. The definition of the product and geographical markets, and the subsequent estimation of market share and concentration cut-off points, are left largely in the hands of the Regional Offices, who are given some benchmarks but have to use their 'judgement of the size of the market' in most cases (p17). There is an ongoing debate in the literature (and in the USA courts) about how to define the relevant market in healthcare, and rather than entering into this debate the guidance, perhaps sensibly, adopts a simple approach based on likely data availability. Nevertheless, even the use of distance and location-based measures faces many difficult methodological issues (see Werden, 1989; Luft and Maerki, 1984; Dranove and Shanley, 1990; Luft et al, 1990; Phelps, 1990). Furthermore, although this approach may be simpler, leaving open the issue of how to define the relevant market allows a great deal of discretion which may be used to produce the 'desired' results from the assessment process. Experience in hospital-merger cases in the USA illustrates that the definitions and indices used can have a major

impact on the conclusions drawn about the impact of merger on competition. In practice, many decisions would have been reversed had slightly different definitions of markets been used (Wilder and Jacobs, 1987; Blackstone and Fuhr, 1989).

Similarly, there is very little detail included on what type of evidence should be accepted as proof of the offsetting benefits from merger. For example, on efficiency gains, the guidance notes the lack of good research evidence on the existence of economies of scale and scope, but does not say what sort of evidence *is* therefore acceptable. In hospital merger cases in the USA, the Justice Department has often ruled out alleged efficiency gains as insufficiently convincing, speculative or insubstantial (Horoschak, 1993), and requires them to be well-documented and specific rather than related to general reductions in overheads or management costs. In addition, it is essential to establish that the gains will be passed on in the form of reduced prices; and that they could not be achieved through a route other than merger. Similarly, claims for improved quality of care receive little weight in the US process as they are less amenable to quantification and authentication (Whitesell and Whitesell, 1995). Even greater problems arise in the assessment of collusive behaviour, as the judgement about whether an action is to be interpreted as co-operative or collusive is even less likely to be supported by hard evidence.

Whilst it may not be appropriate in the NHS to have a policy based on strict rules in which only measurable factors are allowed to influence the decision, some tightening of the 'allowable' evidence would make the process less discretionary (thus giving a greater degree of certainty to those involved) and also avoid wasted effort on the part of those making proposals, who could avoid collecting evidence which will be given little weight in the assessment process.

A further discretionary aspect of regulatory policy is the lack of detail about how decisions should be made when evidence conflicts. For example, the merger policy requires any detrimental impact on competition to be weighed against possible economic and non-economic benefits, but apart from the general statement that the economic benefits should receive 'more' weight than the non-economic ones, no guidance is given on how trade-offs should be made in practice. Although this may reflect the belief that each case is unique, this again allows a great deal of discretion. Indeed, the nature of some of the non-economic benefits suggest that in particular circumstances, mergers are *always* likely to be allowed: for example, where mergers are an alternative to closure, then one of the non-economic benefits includes consideration of the implications of closure of a unit which is 'popular with the public'. As even the most poorly performing hospital is likely to be popular (at least with the local population) when suggestions for closure are made, then unless limits are placed on the weight to be given to this factor, mergers are always likely to be approved in these circumstances. Feedback from Regional Offices involved in implementing merger policy (details of the survey are given in Chapter 6) suggests that 'local circumstances' will always need to be considered as part of the assessment and these may override any criteria set out in national policy.

Similar issues arise in general Competition Law as the MMC judges a merger on the public interest criterion, which requires weighing up the impact on competition against the possible offsetting efficiency gains from merger plus the non-economic factors. One of the main differences is that, in contrast to the MMC, the burden of proof in the NHS guidance rests with the merging parties. The merger is allowed to go ahead only if it has no effect on competition or if the negative effects are outweighed by efficiency or other gains, producing a net benefit overall (p19). In theory at least, this produces a much tougher test for the merger than general competition policy.

The discretionary nature of much of the regulatory policy in the NHS mirrors the regulation of the privatised utilities where it has been noted that 'regulation is evolving into an informal system of rule-making which operates through negotiation and bargaining in the shadow of the law' (Veljanovski, 1991). This is in contrast to regulation in the USA, which tends to be tighter, to follow explicit rules and to be carried out openly with opportunities for

third parties to take part in decision-making (Vogel, 1986). That policy in the UK has taken such a course is perhaps not surprising, as it depends to a large degree on the sort of economic, political and institutional factors facing the industries and their regulators. Where the costs of using informal negotiation and co-operation are low (and the weak accountability of regulators and weak judicial review process suggest this is the case), the regulators will prefer to use such strategies rather than resorting to the legal system (Veljanovski, 1991; Stelzer, 1991).

The discretionary nature of regulatory policy is not necessarily 'bad' per se as it avoids many of the costly and time-consuming processes which can take many years to complete, leaving all parties in a state of uncertainty in the interim. However, it does have some implications for the issue of 'regulatory capture'.

7.5.2 The scope for regulatory capture

Although much of regulatory theory focuses on the way in which regulators carry out the duties assigned to them by Government, there is wide recognition that it is unrealistic to assume that the regulator is always able or willing to act as a perfect agent in terms of having benevolent objectives and acting in the public interest. The danger of 'regulatory capture', in which the regulator acts in the interests of the firms it is regulating, rather than on behalf of the consumer or potential new firms, has been widely discussed (e.g. Stigler, 1971; Peltzman 1976). Technical explanations can be found elsewhere (e.g. Laffont & Tirole, 1993), but in general terms the issue concerns the extent to which regulators over time begin to share the interests of those they regulate, and become 'the victims of their own zeal by failing to maintain an arm's length relationship from the industry' (Veljanovski, 1991).

Particular features of the regulatory system tend to increase the likelihood that regulatory capture will occur, and the extent to which policy is discretionary will have a major influence. For example, if the regulators have a high degree of discretion in interpreting information brought before them, then they are likely to defend vigorously any decisions they take based on their interpretation if subsequently challenged by other authorities. Despite the presence of many conditions which create the potential for regulatory capture, there is no compelling evidence that this has occurred in the privatised utilities to date (Armstrong et al, 1995).

However, the potential for regulatory capture is particularly great in the NHS as not only is policy very discretionary, but the regulators are in an unusual position. Unlike the independent bodies created for the privatised utilities, the Department of Health has given most responsibility for the implementation of regulatory policy to the Regional Offices or to the NHS Executive itself. Regional Offices are often expected to ensure that 'problems' do not arise in their geographical areas, and if this can be achieved through applying regulatory policy in a particular way, the Regional Offices may indeed find it difficult to resist capture. As the guidance places particular emphasis in almost every decision-making process on the role of the regional 'policy board member',[13] this also suggests that political considerations may influence the actions of the regulators.

In summary, although there may well be a danger of regulatory capture, the introduction of a more explicit decision-making framework is likely to have some beneficial impact, as decisions on every aspect of the guidance were previously being undertaken anyway by staff in Regional Offices and NHS Executive headquarters. The introduction of clearer responsibilities and decision criteria may help to eliminate some of the pitfalls associated with regulatory capture.

7.5.3 Interaction with other policies

Regulatory regimes should be designed to complement other policy instruments rather than existing in isolation or even working against other aspects of the policy environment. Given the highly managed nature of the NHS market, there is potential for clashes in policy to occur, and two of the more con-

tentious areas are the policy on promoting new entry, and the financial regime for Trusts.

Policies to promote entry

The potential for new entry influences the extent to which a market is contestable and is highlighted in the merger guidance as one of the factors to be taken into account in estimating the impact on competition. Dawson has criticised the UK merger guidelines for not recognising the limits which Trusts face on their ability to enter the market by supplying new services, and has argued that most entry would therefore come from the private sector (Dawson, 1995). It is argued that the regulations which apply to access capital funds by Trusts will limit the extent to which they can compete for market share, other than in temporary ways by using spare capacity to attract extra demand (e.g. from waiting list initiatives). For the signal from a potential supplier to be credible, Dawson argues that capital commitment is usually required, and as access to public funding for capital (beyond a minimum level) is centrally controlled, it is unlikely that the Department of Health will allow Trusts to borrow capital in order to mount a threat to an incumbent Trust in another location.[14] Private sector suppliers would face no such barriers, but are likely to 'cherry-pick' in order to provide only those services in which they perceive strong potential for profits.

It is likely that this underestimates the potential for Trusts to compete in terms of new entry, as there are some services for which access to capital will not be required in order to compete. Also, for many Trusts, especially those in urban areas where spare capacity of capital is unlikely to be temporary and can be dealt with either by selling buildings or by using them to develop and expand new services, entry into different markets may be possible. In the latter case, it may be more difficult to find the non-capital inputs needed to set up a service. Nevertheless, where substantial new capital is required, it is true that the need to fulfil the requirements of the Department of Health and Treasury in order to gain access to public capital funding does indeed provide a barrier to Trusts wishing to develop new services. The central administration of capital resources is aimed not only at ensuring consistency in the allocation of funds, but also avoiding duplication which would be seen as wasting public funds. Similar arguments have been put forward in the USA, where Certificate of Need laws exist in most states in an attempt to avoid duplication of facilities and over-supply of beds. Commentators have highlighted the tension between such laws and the focus on competition which is embodied in the merger guidelines (Kopit and McCann, 1988).

There is a dichotomy here between a competitive process which requires entry and exit, which in the NHS is regulated, and ongoing competition, which requires excess capacity, which may be seen as wasteful. This distinction between competition *for* the market and competition *in* the market is recognised in the NHS guidance, which notes that in some circumstances, it may be more efficient to have only one provider in the market at a time, but that the market should at least be contestable. This suggests that although there may well be monopoly in the *provision* of facilities, there can potentially be contestability in the *operation* of services. Regulatory policy in other sectors has recognised this distinction. For example, in the telecommunications industry, following a review of the initial decision to permit only a single entrant (Mercury), access to British Telecom's networks is now much more open and entry into the mobile phone and apparatus sector has also improved. Similarly, privatisation of the railways has taken the form of maintaining monopolies in provision of the tracks whilst franchising the operation of services to other suppliers through a competitive process.

This suggests that the role of entry or threat of entry could be enhanced by the Department of Health, without the need to alter the restrictions on access to capital, if the ownership and operation of assets in the NHS were clearly separated. For example, a purchaser who is dissatisfied with the way in which the A&E service is being provided at the local hospital has little leverage as a competing A&E service is not feasible. However, if it were possible to force the incumbent provider to lease or rent the assets associated with the A&E service to another Trust (if poor management is the problem) or to allow alternative groups of doctors to use the assets (if clinical quality is an issue), then entry would be effectively facilitated. Indeed, this could in theory apply at all levels, from access to a single machine or operating theatre to access to the total assets of the Trust. Although the Department of Health suggests this course of action itself (in a rather guarded manner), not within the guidance on mergers, but in the section on managing Trusts in difficulty,[15] and although there is no legal impediment to this separation as the Secretary of State ultimately owns all assets, strong professional and practical barriers make this a difficult practical option.

Whilst there are some examples of this sort of arrangement in the NHS at present (e.g. where one Trust might allow doctors from other Trusts to use facilities), these appear to be restricted to cases where all parties are gaining from the arrangement and enter into it willingly. It would clearly be far more difficult to achieve if the incumbent Trust was losing business and was an unwilling party. Professional ties amongst groups of medical staff would also make it difficult for Trusts to gain co-operation for such ventures. Recently, one Trust in Scotland appeared to be close to losing the whole management board, creating a possible precedent for future actions (Health Services Journal, 23 January 1997).

In summary, there is some potential, even within the existing structures, for increasing the extent to which entry and the threat of entry could be used as a method of enhancing competition in the NHS, and this would reduce the extent to which different aspects of the current regime work in opposition to each other.

Financial regime for Trusts

It could be argued that as NHS Trusts are forced to follow the pricing and costing rules and are not free to make profits to use as they wish, regulatory policy aimed at preventing market power is misguided as Trusts have no incentive to exercise this power by charging higher prices in order to reap the gains (Craig and Forbes, 1996). This is certainly an argument heard in relation to non-profit-making hospitals in the USA, where some have argued that the anti-trust policy is far less relevant to these organisations owing to the nature of their pricing policy (Kopit and McCann, 1988). However, these views are misguided as in addition to the dead-weight welfare losses associated with monopoly profits, firms with market power may face very little incentive to reduce costs by using their resources efficiently and may also be slow to innovate and respond to customers. Indeed, one of the greatest benefits for the monopolist is said to be a 'quiet life' (Vickers and Hay, 1987). Implementing cost-saving mechanisms is likely to involve considerable time and effort on the part of Trusts and may cause problems in keeping staff motivated. If Trusts can avoid these activities by virtue of their market power, they can pass increased costs onto their purchasers. Experience in the USA suggests that anti-trust authorities are often even *more* concerned about the impact of market power of non-profit-making hospitals than about the impact of their profit-making counterparts, as the former will have less incentive to reduce costs in order to reap higher profits (Vistnes, 1995).

Price regulation has been a major responsibility of the regulators of the privatised utilities, and the RPI-X method of price capping has been adopted widely. In contrast to the traditional rate of return regulation which has been used extensively in the USA, the UK has opted for regulation of price rather than profit, by fixing price increases for a defined basket of goods or services in line with the level of inflation (retail price index) minus an allowance for productivity increases ('X'), where X is set for a number of years in advance. The economic arguments for the superiority of price over rate of return regulation cannot be considered in detail here (see Vickers and Yarrow, 1989, for details), but relate to the incentives faced by the regulated firms and the cost of administering the system. Rate of return regulation allows higher costs to be passed through to the consumer, providing little incentive for firms to keep costs low. Meanwhile, price caps encourage productive efficiency as firms can retain

the fruits of this productivity by reaping higher profits until the next price review. This also provides an incentive for innovation and technological progress (where these reduce costs). Furthermore, the calculation of price indices is much simpler than the alternatives under rate of return regulation, which require calculation of the asset base and estimates of future costs and demand.

In the UK the price-cap method is intended to lighten the burden of regulation, because once X has been set in advance for a period of around five years (long enough to give the firm an incentive to reduce costs so they can retain profits, but short enough to allow the regulator to take into account potential for future efficiency gains), the regulator does not need to interfere with the firm's pricing or investment behaviour. Additionally, the process is explicit and non-discretionary. Although in theory the price-cap method ignores the levels of profit made by firms during the five-year period for which X is set, in practice there has been pressure for the regulators to act on the perceived excessive profits made in some industries. For example, in the first five years of BT's privatisation, OFTEL threatened at least three times to revise the formula in the light of BT's 'high' profitability (Veljanovski, 1991), and there has been recent controversy over Littlechild's decision to reset X in order to reduce the prices charged in the electricity industry.

At present, the pricing regime in the NHS incorporates the drawbacks of rate of return regulation in terms of the passing-on of higher costs, but unlike other industries, Trusts also face regulation of profits in the form of restrictions on their rate of return. It has been suggested that the NHS might move towards a price-cap method if the need for price regulation continued (Propper, 1995). The recent review of the Trust financial regime considered the pros and cons of moving to a price-cap method, possibly only in sectors where monopoly power is most likely to be held (e.g. emergency services), but ultimately rejected this on the grounds that it was 'inappropriate and difficult to implement' in healthcare (NHS Executive 1996, p50). However, the suggestions for liberalisation of the Trust regime imply that the regulatory regime may still need to tackle the issue of monopoly pricing and profits in the future.

7.6 THE FUTURE DIRECTION OF REGULATORY POLICY

7.6.1 Changes within the existing framework

Existing economic regulatory policy addresses some of the issues related to concentration of services, largely by attempting to promote a competitive structure on the supply side and through the regulation of some aspects of conduct. However, it tends to be highly discretionary, raising issues of regulatory capture, with some elements unlikely to operate in the same direction as other central policies. These issues could be addressed to some extent by amending the existing guidance in several ways. In order to clarify the use of the guidance and to help achieve consistency in application, the following would be useful:

- greater detail about the potential sources of data for collecting evidence at each step of proposed mergers and Trust viability assessments;
- more precise definitions of key components of the policy, such as measures of the relevant 'market';
- guidance on the sort of evidence which is considered valid, especially in relation to efficiency benefits, quality gains and potential for new entry;
- a more explicit method of weighting the various components of the assessment, although clearly this would not be straightforward. In particular, one point arising from the Regional Office survey was the need to recognise the political context in which local decisions are made.

The aim is not to produce a 'rule book' which is followed mechanistically, but to reduce the extent to which the assessment methods are used in a discretionary manner. Additionally, one response from the Regional Office survey noted that the cost of undertaking the level of

analysis required by the assessments was prohibitive. Greater detail and clarity of guidance on the key elements of the policy (for example, how to define the 'market') would therefore also have the effect of reducing the input required from the Regional Office and from other parties, perhaps providing a greater incentive to put the policies into action.

Regulatory policy might also be amended to reflect better the context in which it is applied. In particular, policy on mergers should acknowledge the full range of driving forces for merger (which have been discussed in Chapter 6), rather than being focused largely on issues related to economies of scale and scope. If mergers are being driven by central policies on training, professional recommendations on service delivery, the need to reduce spare capacity and many other factors, these need to be incorporated into the assessment process in some way in order to make policy relevant to specific circumstances. This would also allow more explicit consideration of the role of merger in relation to a 'failing' Trust and the need to be clear about the source of this failure before deciding that merger is necessarily an appropriate solution. Given the uncertainties about the level and source of the potential benefits from the concentration of services, a requirement to undertake post-merger analysis is also an essential addition to current policy. This should incorporate estimates of the extent to which efficiency gains were achieved and the subsequent impact on costs, prices and quality.

Further consideration should be given to the way in which regulatory policy aimed at encouraging competition fits with existing policy on pricing and entry. There are signs that the Department of Health recognises that aspects of the current Trust financial regime may need to be amended (NHS Executive 1996), and if such developments go ahead, the regulation of prices in order to prevent abuse of monopoly power will require further attention.

Finally, a thorough review of how the policy has been implemented to date and of the way in which the assessments have been undertaken, including the interpretation and weighting of each element in the assessment process and the subsequent decision, would provide a basis for making the amendments suggested above. Without this knowledge it is difficult to assess exactly how regulatory policy might be improved.

7.6.2 New directions

Regulatory policy targeted at the supply side of the healthcare market will also be influenced by changes occurring on the demand side. Purchasers may use countervailing monopoly power to offset the potential for the exercise of monopoly power by providers. As Dawson notes (1995), the US experience with managed care illustrated how the emergence of large, strong purchasers through the growth of managed care had a significant impact on costs and prices (the relevant literature is summarised in Goddard and Ferguson, 1997). GP fundholding *could* be interpreted as a fragmentation of the purchasing function which may allow monopoly providers to exploit their position far more in relationships with fundholders, whose purchases account for a much smaller proportion of income for a Trust, than with the larger commissioning authorities. However, the development of consortia and multi-funds in which contracts are set on behalf of all fundholders in the group has enhanced the market and negotiating power of fundholders, and in the UK there are currently at least 16 multifunds covering over three million patients (Mays and Dixon 1996). Indeed, Trusts appear remarkably keen to keep even individual fundholders happy, and although early evidence suggested that fundholders were willing to switch between providers (usually on quality grounds) (Glennerster et al, 1994; Mahon et al, 1994), a more recent Audit Commission survey suggested that the majority of fundholders have made no major changes to where they refer (Audit Commission, 1996).

The shape of purchasing may change yet again under Labour Government plans and it is possible that the leverage of purchasers will be enhanced further, both through the merger of Health Authorities to create fewer but larger purchasers, and through the creation of local commissioning groups to include all GPs working in co-operation with Health Authorities (Labour Party, 1996).[16] Thus regulatory policy could be re-directed to encourage the development of purchaser power, not necessarily or solely in terms of size, but also, for example, by improving the availability and quality of information on which purchasing decisions are made, rather than by attempting to control monopoly on the supply side. The UK regulatory guidance does indeed contain a section on purchaser merger, but the focus is largely on ensuring that larger purchasing organisations remain sensitive and responsive to their population (i.e. on the nature of the agency relationship between consumers and purchasers), rather than on their bargaining power in relation to monopoly providers.

Regulatory policy may also take a new direction if the separation of the ownership and operation of Trusts' assets and facilities is given serious consideration. In this case, regulation would not be aimed at controlling the concentration of services through merger policy, but instead would be focused on providing a competitive process for access to facilities by the operators, perhaps through a franchise system as suggested by Propper (1995). The 'franchise operators' might be management or clinical teams, or a combination of both. The franchise terms would need to be set by the regulator, and this would include: (a) decisions on the duration of the franchise, which would have an important influence on the incentives to invest in the assets; (b) aspects of service delivery such as minimum quality standards, clinical effectiveness and prices; and (c) the terms under which the franchise agreement could be terminated early. The regulator would also need to organise the award of franchises by arranging the bidding process. The separation of ownership and operation of assets would of course be made much sharper if hospital assets were owned by the private sector, although this might prove to be politically unpopular.

The question of *who* should undertake the regulatory function is likely to arise in the future. Some commentators have already suggested that the dangers of regulatory capture of the Regional Offices are so great that the NHS should follow the example of the privatised utilities and set up an independent regulator such as 'OFHEALTH' (Propper, 1995). However, this would not guarantee that regulatory capture would be avoided. Such an arrangement also does not take into account the difficulties of operating a separate system alongside the many other regulatory functions carried out by the Department of Health. Regulators for the privatised utilities tend to have responsibility across a whole range of factors such as setting minimum quality standards, pricing, profits, capital and approval of licences to operate services. In the NHS, it is unlikely to be appropriate to have an independent body carrying out *all* these regulatory functions, which raises the question of the respective roles and responsibilities of the NHS Executive and a body such as 'OFHEALTH'.

An alternative might be to shift regulatory responsibilities from the regional tier to other parts of the NHS. The expansion of fundholding and the development of a primary care-led NHS has already marked a new strategic role for Health Authorities, with some regulatory responsibilities. The Labour Party's proposals suggest an even greater role for GPs in direct purchasing, again emphasising the strategic commissioning role and performance management responsibilities of the Health Authorities and suggesting that they might merge and take on a 'semi-regional as well as a district role' (Labour Party, 1996). Thus, it is possible that in the future Health Authorities will be responsible for implementing regulatory policy, either in their current form or as substitutes for the regional tier. Clearly, Health Authorities can be expected to have access to a greater range of relevant local information and intelligence which is essential to the regulatory function, and thus decision-making may well be improved. Nevertheless, it would be misleading to assume that devolution of such responsibilities would necessarily reduce the likelihood of regulatory capture. Indeed, as Health Authorities will often have formed close relationships with local Trusts and may be directly affected by decisions on issues such as Trust mergers, they are potentially even more likely to be susceptible to influence over the desired outcome than the more distant regional tier. If, however, Health Authorities are assumed to be the closest 'agents' for their resident populations, it is more possible to conflate the objectives of the regulator with those of the public interest.

7.7 CONCLUSIONS

The nature and role of regulatory policy in relation to the concentration of healthcare services in the NHS have been reviewed, with reference to approaches taken in other sectors with similar market characteristics. The discretionary nature of policy in the NHS has been highlighted, together with the areas in which it clashes with other aspects of central policy. If the Department of Health is to formulate a consistent regulatory policy for the NHS, it is necessary to acknowledge the potential for different policies to work in opposing directions and to address this explicitly. In view of this, suggestions have been made for the future direction of policy, both in terms of adjusting policy within the existing regulatory framework and in terms of taking policy forward in new directions. Consideration should be given to reviewing the degree of success with which existing regulatory policy has been applied, and to the issue of who should be responsible for implementation at local level in the future.

REFERENCES

Armstrong M, Cowen S, Vickers J 1995 Regulatory Reform. Economic Analysis and British Experience. MIT Press, Cambridge, Massachusetts.
Audit Commission 1996 What the Doctor Ordered. Audit Commission, London.
Bain J 1956 Barriers to New Competition. Harvard University Press, Cambridge, Massachusetts.

Baumol W J, Panzar J C, Willig R D 1982 Contestable Markets and the Theory of Industry Structure. Harcourt, Brace and Jovanovich, New York.
Blackorby C, Donaldson D, Weymark J A 1982 A Normative Approach to Industrial Performance Evaluation and Concentration Indices. European Economic Review 19:89-121.

Blackstone E A, Fuhr J P 1989 Hospital Mergers and Antitrust: An Economic Analysis. Journal of Health Politics, Policy and Law 14:383-403.

Craig N, Forbes J 1996 Blind Choice or Informed faith? Cognitive Dissonance and Competition in Health Care. Paper to Health Economists Study Group, January, 1996.

Dawson D 1995 Regulating Competition in the NHS: The Department of Health Guide on Mergers and Anti-Competitive Behaviour. University of York Discussion Paper 131, York.

Demsetz H 1973 Industry Structure, Market Rivalry and Public Policy. Journal of Law and Economics 16:1–9

Department of Health 1993 Making London Better. HMSO, London.

Department of Justice & Federal Trade Commission (DOJ/FTC) 1992 Statement Accompanying Release of Revised Merger Guidelines. April 2 1992, Washington.

Donsimoni M-P, Geroski P, Jacquemin A 1984 Concentration Indices and Market Power ; Two Views. The Journal of Industrial Economics 32:419–434.

Dranove D, Shanley M 1990 A Note on the Relational Aspects of Hospital Market Definitions. Journal of Health Economics 8:473–478.

Ferguson P R, Ferguson G J 1994 Industrial Economics: Issues and Perspectives. Macmillan, Basingstoke.

Glennerster H, Matsaganis M, Owens P, Hancock S 1994 GP Fundholding: Wild Card or Winning Hand? In Robinson and Le Grand 1994.

Goddard M, Ferguson B 1997 Mergers in the NHS : Made in Heaven or Marriages of Convenience? Nuffield Provincial Hospitals Trust Occasional Paper (forthcoming).

Health Services Journal 1996 That Sinking Feeling. 26 September: 11.

Health Services Journal 1997 Scots Missed? 23 January: 15

Horoschak M J 1993 An Overview of the Federal Trade Commission's Health Care Antitrust Program. United States of America Federal Trade Commission, Washington DC.

Jacquemin A 1987 The New Industrial Organisation. Clarendon Press, Oxford.

Kirzner I 1973 Competition and Entrepreneurship. University of Chicago Press, Chicago.

Kopit W G, McCann R W 1988 Toward a Definitive Antitrust Standard for Nonprofit Hospital Mergers. Journal of Health Politics, Policy and Law 13:635–662.

KPMG Management Consulting 1996 Review of the Trust Finance Regime – an Analysis of the Cost Equals Price Survey Results. KPMG report to NHS Executive.

Labour Party 1996 A Health Service for a New Century. Speech given by Chris Smith MP, 3 December 1996.

Laffont J J, Tirole J 1993 A Theory of Incentives in Procurement and Regulation. MIT Press, Cambridge.

Le Grand J, Bartlett W (eds) 1993 Quasi-Markets and Social Policy. Macmillan, Basingstoke.

Luft H and Maerki S 1984 Competitive Potential of Hospitals and their Neighbours. Contemporary Policy Issues 3:89–102.

Luft H, Phibbs C S, Garnick D W, Robinson J C 1990 Rejoinder to Dranove and Shanley. Journal of Health Economics, 8:479–83.

Mahon A, Wilkin D, Whitehouse C 1994 Choice of Hospital for Elective Surgery Referrals: GPs' and Patients' Views, in Robinson and Le Grand 1994.

Mays N , Dixon J 1996 Purchaser Plurality in UK Health Care. Kings Fund, London.

Mueller D C 1996 Lessons from the United State's Antitrust History. International Journal of Industrial Organisation, 14:415–445

NHS Executive 1994 The Operation of the NHS Internal Market: Local Freedoms, National Responsibilities (HSG(94)55). HMSO, London.

NHS Executive 1996 Review of the Trust Financial Regime. HMSO, London

NHS Management Executive 1993 Costing for Contracting (FDL(93)51). HMSO, London.

Norman G, La Manna M (eds) 1992 The New Industrial Economics. Recent Developments in Industrial Organisation, Oligopoly and Game Theory. Edward Elgar, England.

Peltzman S 1976 Towards a More General Theory of Regulation. Journal of Law and Economics 14:109–48.

Phelps C E 1990 A Welfare-Based Approach to Analysing Markets and Mergers. Journal of Health Economics 8:464–72.

Propper C 1995 Regulatory Reform of the NHS Internal Market. Health Economics 4:77–83.

Robinson R, Le Grand J (eds) 1994 Evaluating the NHS Reforms. King's Fund, London.

Shepherd W 1995 Contestability versus Competition – Once More. Land Economics 71:200–309

Stelzer I M 1991 Regulatory Methods : A Case for Hands Across the Atlantic. In Veljanovski 1991.

Stigler G 1971 The Theory of Economic Regulation. Bell Journal of Economics 2:3–21.

Tomlinson B 1992 Report of the Inquiry into London's Health Service, Medical Education and Research. HMSO, London.

Veljanovski C 1991 The Regulation Game in Veljanovski C (ed) Regulators and the Market : An Assessment of the Growth of Regulation in the UK. Institute of Economic Affairs, London.

Vickers J, Hay D 1987 The Economics of Market Dominance. The Economics of Market Dominance (eds) Hay D and Vickers J, Blackwell, Oxford.

Vickers J, Yarrow G 1989 Privatisation: An Economic Analysis. MIT Press, London.

Vistnes G 1995 Hospital Mergers and Antitrust Enforcement. Journal of Health Politics, Policy and Law 20:175–190.

Vogel D 1986 National Styles of Regulation. Cornell University Press, New York.

Werden G J 1989 The Limited Relevance of Patient Migration Data in Market Delineation for Hospital Merger Cases. Journal of Health Economics 8:363–376.

Whitesell S E, Whitesell W E 1995 Hospital Mergers and Antitrust: Some Economic and Legal Issues. American Journal of Economics and Sociology 5:305–21.

Wilder R P, Jacobs P 1987 Antitrust Considerations for Hospital Mergers: Market Definition and Market Concentration. Advances in Health Economics and Health Services Research 7:245–262.

Williams M E 1993 The Effectiveness of Competition Policy in the United Kingdom. Oxford Review of Economic Policy 9:94–112.

Williamson O E 1985 The Economic Institutions of Capitalism. Free Press, New York.

Williamson O E 1989 Transaction Cost Economics. In R Schmalensee & R Willig (eds) Handbook of Industrial Organisation Volume 1. North-Holland, Amsterdam.

NOTES

1 The restrictive nature of the assumptions around the manner and cost of entry which are at the heart of the theory of contestable markets has been debated and discussed for many years (e.g. Shepherd, 1995) and it is widely recognised that the conditions for perfect contestability are unlikely to occur in practice. However, the strength of this approach was to recognise that factors other than the degree of market concentration influence the exercise of market power.

2 Whilst the range of potential outcomes from the 'games' which firms may play offer insights into the way in which markets may work, this also limits the predictive ability of the models, making it difficult to draw policy implications.

3 There are several other elements in the Austrian critique of traditional theory which cannot be considered in detail here, but involve the implications of partial rather than perfect knowledge on the actions of economic agents and a move away from a focus on equilibrium states to the continual flux of the competitive process.

4 For example, treatment of vertical restraints (see Mueller, 1996; Vickers and Hay, 1987).

5 There were undoubtedly also political imperatives for putting regulatory structures into place.

6 Where the production level corresponding to the lowest unit cost of the firm is sufficient to satisfy all demand when price is set at that cost – in other words, where the nature of production makes it most efficient to have just a single firm operating in a market.

7 Other market failures which are also relevant for regulation concern asymmetric information and problems of externalities (see Armstrong et al, 1995, for discussion).

8 In the following discussion, the focus is on economic regulation rather than on the many other types of regulation which characterise the NHS – for example, management relationships between purchasers and the NHS Executive; public accountability and probity of NHS Trusts; professional self-regulation; consumer complaints procedures and national quality targets (such as the Patients' Charter).

9 Despite the lack of strong research evidence to support this, as illustrated in previous chapters.

10 The guidelines do not advocate the use of an index, probably because the data required to construct such indices are not generally available. Most indices have some drawbacks (Donsimoni et al, 1984; Blackorby et al, 1982), but the USA antitrust guidelines which are applied to the healthcare sector advocate the Herfindahl–Hirschman Index (HHI) as a measure of concentration in hospital markets (DOJ/FTC, 1992).

11 These include the limited choice of providers of some services (e.g. emergency services where access is key) in some areas (e.g. rural locations with a single provider); the nature of the pricing regime which means that providers left with large fixed costs following the loss of a contract will need to add these on to the price of remaining services as all costs must be recouped, thus providing a disincentive for purchasers to shift business if they end up indirectly footing the bill through payment for other services; thirdly, closures and major downsizing are not politically palatable.

12 The difference between the amount of capital spending agreed for a Trust and the amount they have generated internally. Trusts are not allowed to exceed the limit set, but if they undershoot they can carry forward spending power to the following year.

13 The selection of regional policy board members requires approval from the Secretary of State for Health.

14 The Conservative Government perceived a smaller role for public sector funding of capital developments in the NHS in the future, but at present it is not clear how widespread the use of private sector-funds will be as major projects have been limited.

15 Where it is acknowledged that a Trust may be viable under different management and lists a set of actions to be taken where management appears to be poor (NHS Executive, 1994, p39).

16 Although a Labour Government will of course be stressing the equity advantages of such arrangements rather than the leverage of the purchasing groups.

8

The nature and consequences of provider consolidations in the US

Richard J. Arnould, Lawrence M. DeBrock, Heather L. Radach

8.1 INTRODUCTION

Healthcare reforms in the US have resulted in substantial structural changes in the provider industries. As recently as two decades ago the various components of the provider side of healthcare were totally independent and non-integrated. Most hospitals were free-standing, single-facility enterprises operating as not-for-profit tax-exempt entities. Physicians were largely organized as sole practitioners or in very small single specialty groups.[1] Other types of providers, such as long-term care, laboratory and radiology, were also free-standing entities. Today the provider who has not engaged in some form of horizontal or vertical integration is an anomaly. The types and levels of integration range from horizontal integration within a provider type and market to completely diversified community-care networks that contain all types of providers and may even be extended to insurers. Levels of contractual integration within these structural forms of integration range from short-term contractual ties to complete financial integration.

Much attention is being directed by researchers and policy-makers to important issues related to these structural changes. The first important issue is to identify the economic forces within the policy changes that are bringing about incentives for horizontal and vertical integration among healthcare providers. The second issue is to determine the economic effects of these structural changes. The third is to determine if the economic effects are consistent with the outcomes that were sought by the changes in policies that originally led to the structural changes.

In this chapter we attempt to provide a basis for understanding the structural changes that have occurred in the US. While our general discussion relates to all types of integration, we concentrate our detailed descriptions of events on hospital mergers and consolidations. Before looking directly at the hospital industry, we will outline the impact of managed care on the US healthcare industry by looking at the history of competition and competitive reforms. Second, we will closely examine the benefits of competition and managed care. This examination will lead to studies of hospital competition and the behaviour of markets with varying levels of competition. Third, we will present a history of the market structure in the hospital industry focusing on the large number of mergers occurring in the last 20 years. This naturally leads into an examination of the effect mergers have on hospital services, which will focus specifically on efficiency, price and cost issues. Finally, we will examine how antitrust litigation, both actual and threatened, figure into the analysis and impact upon the incentives of hospitals and the industry as a whole. The conclusion then will begin to ask the questions which should be addressed in the future.

8.2 COMPETITIVE REFORMS IN THE US HEALTHCARE SYSTEM

There has been much emphasis on health-policy reform in the US since the mid-1980s due to two significant problems – costs and access. Costs of medical care in the US have been increasing at an alarming rate for two to three decades. Healthcare expenditures represented approximately 7 per cent of GDP in 1969, but had grown to 14 per cent by the early 1990s (National Center for Health Services Statistics, 1992). The US Congressional Bureau of the Budget (1992) forecasted that it would reach 18 per cent of GDP by the year 2000 if not brought under control.

The US has a private and public health-insurance system. Most employed people in the US under the age of 65 are covered by some form of private insurance. There are two major public insurance products: Medicare provides coverage for those over 65 and for other limited populations; Medicaid provides medical coverage for certain of the poor who qualify. In spite of the rapid increase in expenditures in healthcare and the extensive insurance system, an estimated 33 million people in the US have no public or private insurance coverage. An additional segment of the population is underinsured. Approximately 1 in 7 of those under 65 are uninsured (US Congressional Budget Office, 1992). Those who are uninsured have limited access to healthcare providers. Hospitals are legally required to provide care to anyone who appears at their door in a life-threatening condition. However, access often is not convenient for the poor and uninsured, and this results in their seeking care at a time when their health condition is more mature and more costly to treat.

Certain institutional factors present in the US healthcare system provided the economic incentives that fuelled the problems of costs and access. The private insurance system in the US is tied to employment, i.e. it is provided in part or total through an arrangement between employer and employee as a benefit. Health insurance generally had its inception as an employee benefit in the 1940s and 1950s. Following WWII there were wage freezes and it was during this time that bargaining groups concentrated on increasing benefits to workers. As a result, health-insurance benefits grew rapidly. The growth in health-insurance was fuelled by the tax treatment of health-insurance premiums, which were considered a deductible business ex-pense for employers and non-taxable income for recipients.

The nature of the insurance products that emerged further provided perverse incentives for producers, consumers and insurers in a classic principal–agent setting with asymmetric information. Both consumers and employers found they could purchase superior coverage or receive lower rates if healthy individuals were placed in smaller rating groups. This obviously resulted in adverse selection and could only be maintained if insurance contracts contained restrictions on the portability (from one insurer to another) of an existing condition. Access became a problem for anyone who wished to change employment but had a pre-existing condition.

Inflation was most certainly built into the insurance products because most providers were reimbursed on a retrospective fee-for-service basis and the insureds received service benefits coverage. Providers had incentives to provide excessive levels of service so long as the payment for those services exceeded their marginal disutility from the loss of leisure. Patients and insurers found it difficult to monitor the appropriateness of the level of care being delivered. Patients had little reason to seek efficient providers as a result of the tax benefits. Thus, moral hazard resulted and took the form of providing excessive levels of care, each unit of which was not necessarily produced efficiently. Price of services was effectively eliminated as a dimension over which providers competed and was replaced by a very costly form of quality competition. Quality competition generated extensive excess capacity of costly forms of technology and an excessive reliance on medical specialists. Most patients could request any level of treatment. Furthermore, patients had direct access to virtually any level of specialist.

It is important to recognise certain institutional factors in that existed in the US healthcare system prior to competitive reforms. Both the private and public insurance systems relied almost entirely on private, market-oriented delivery systems. Reliance on the market in the US healthcare system is often considered to be a recent occurrence. This certainly is not supported by the facts. Also, analysts of the system often point to competitive reforms as bringing about some first-time recognition that the US system is driven by economic incentives. Certainly, the prevailing tax and insurance system contained economic incentives, which generated behaviour by providers and patients consistent with the economic behaviour that would be predicted by economic models. That system generated problems because the underlying incentives were not compatible with efficient outcomes.

A second feature of US healthcare system, both before and after competitive reforms, is heavy regulation. It was regulated before the reforms were enacted. It continues to be heavily regulated. The reforms did not bring about free, unregulated healthcare markets. Quality, entry, and virtually every other aspect of every type of healthcare provider is regulated in some fashion.

Finally, reforms initially were driven by the private sector's desire to find ways to reduce the growing cost of the healthcare benefit to employers, i.e. to contain costs. Independent insurers operated primarily as pass-through agents (Havighurst, 1988) with little desire to bring about cost containment.[2] Large corporations began to self-insure. Once they were bearing significant levels of risk as self-insurers, they sought forms of cost containment that required reforms in the regulatory infrastructure. Public insurers soon followed suit. Generally, the reforms described below permitted the evolution of a variety of forms of managed care which redirected incentives for patients, providers and insurers to seek efficient levels of care.

8.2.1. The nature of competitive reforms[3]

Competitive reforms in the US came from a variety of sources. They are not the result of a single change in laws, although it was necessary to change some laws to permit certain of the reforms to take place. The driving force behind the reforms has been to generate incentives to bring about more efficient consumption and production of healthcare. Dranove (1993) has labelled these reforms as being directed toward patient-driven and payer-driven incentives.

Patient-driven reforms have focused on increasing the level of consumer cost sharing. Levels of coverage contained in standard employer-provided insurance packages declined in the 1970s and 1980s. Frequently, coverage was limited by requiring copayments and deductibles. Copayments and deductibles are intended to increase the incentives for consumers to shop for more efficient providers of insurance products.

Supply-side strategies involved rigorous enforcement of the antitrust laws. For many years healthcare providers enjoyed a limited exemption from the antitrust laws. The relaxation of the exemption of professional services from coverage by the antitrust laws that resulted from a series of Supreme Court decisions in the 1970s has brought about vigorous enforcement to limit the ability of providers to engage in a variety of anti-competitive practices, such as price fixing and hospital mergers, that substantially lessen competition.

Enabling legislation permitted changes in insurance products that generated a number of private-sector initiatives to increase efficiency in the consumption and production of healthcare services. Specifically, this legislation permitted managed-care organisations such as preferred-provider organisations (PPOs) to negotiate prices selectively with providers and to steer patients to efficient vendors. The steering of patients is an important component of payer-driven competitive reforms. Unlike patient-driven competition, payer-driven competitive reforms provide incentives for providers to produce efficient healthcare services and to direct patients under their care to other efficient producers. The incentives are usually provided as a result of prospective pricing arrangements, competitive bidding and risk-sharing contracts with providers.

Competitive reforms are very prevalent in public-sector programmes such as Medicaid. Various states have engaged in different types of competitive reforms. The State of California instituted competitive bidding and selective contracting for services delivered to patients insured under MediCal, the California version of Medicaid. Some other states followed suit. More recently a number of states have begun to use various forms of managed care to provide incentives for the efficient consumption and production of healthcare services delivered to Medicaid patients.

The Federal Government has used the Prospective Payment System and the Resource Based Relative Value Schedule to reimburse hospitals and physicians respectively. These use competitive incentives less directly than the methods described above but do provide incentives for efficient production of services. Where there may be some element of monop-

oly power in the market, prospective prices are a form of 'yardstick competition' (Schleifer, 1985). Using hospitals as an example, the price initially may be based on historic operating costs. However, unlike the cost-plus pricing situations, producer surplus is dependent upon the level of efficiency. If costs are reduced, the producer increases the level of retained surplus. Prospective price levels may be adjusted over time as the levels of retained surplus increase or decrease.

Finally, competitive reforms have been implemented in insurance markets largely by the use of payer and provider-driven incentives described above in a wide variety of private insurance products. The expanded insurance products have focused on generating more competitive insurance products that in turn result in savings from choosing more efficient alternatives. These savings are, at least partially, passed on to consumers.

In summary, it is important to note that most of the reforms that brought change in the incentive systems faced by consumers and producers of healthcare services were not the result of major changes in the laws. The most important changes in laws were those that permitted the steering of patients covered by private and public insurance programmes. They were usually changes in the various states' regulations of health insurance. Without this provision, consumers had no incentive to seek efficient providers, nor did providers risk loss of patients as a result of being high cost. The insurance products through which many of the competitive incentives were delivered generally fit under the rubric of managed care. In the next section, we briefly discuss the nature of managed care in the US and the forces that brought about structural change among providers in the industry.

8.3 BENEFITS FROM MANAGED CARE

Competitive reforms have been implemented largely (but in no way totally) through a variety of forms of managed care. There is no single factor that identifies managed-care systems. Iglehart (1994) has defined managed care as comprising systems that, 'in varying degrees, integrates the financing and delivery of medical care through contracts with selected providers and hospitals that provide comprehensive health services to enrolled members for a predicted monthly premium.' Arnould et al (1993) draw three important components from this and other definitions of managed care. Managed care consists of 'contractual arrangements with selected providers to furnish a comprehensive set of healthcare services to members, usually at negotiated prices... financial incentives to steer patients toward providers and procedures within the plan, and ongoing accountability of providers for their clinical and financial performance.'

The most prevalent forms of managed care in the US are Health Maintenance Organizations (HMOs). HMOs contract with a wide array of providers to deliver comprehensive healthcare services to patient members. Members are required to use HMO providers, i.e. there is 100 per cent copayment for use of providers outside the HMO.[4] Preferred Provider Organizations (PPOs) operate similarly with contractual arrangements with providers, called preferred providers, to furnish comprehensive services to members at pre-negotiated prices. Members have considerable incentives to choose a preferred provider because copayments are substantially lower than when using an out-of-plan administrator. However, members are subject to something less than a 100 per cent copayment in the case of PPOs. Point of Service plans (POSs) are a relatively new form of managed care that are a cross between HMOs and PPOs. Other forms of managed care include utilization review and quality assurance. Throughout this section, we will use HMOs and PPOs to proxy 'managed care'. Christensen et al (1991) provide an excellent discussion of the growth of these entities. Of course, HMOs and PPOs are different forms of managed care. Gold et al (1995) indicate that the typical cost reduction is larger in HMOs than PPOs.

The benefits of a competitive market system are that consumers get the maximum product or service at the lowest price, the service is produced efficiently, producers must respond to consumers' tastes, and economic welfare is maximised.[5] All of these outcomes result from market forces. Certain conditions are necessary for markets to provide this ideal outcome. There must be room in the market for multiple suppliers. Suppliers must act independently of one another. Consumers must be well informed and capable of determining quality, and there must be no production or consumption externalities.

In summary, managed care works to change incentives by forcing participants to pay attention to price and cost attributes, i.e. by making providers and patients more sensitive to the cost of services being provided. The following section considers the empirical findings of such efficiencies.

8.3.1 Evidence of benefits of payer-driven hospital competition

There have been a number of studies documenting the effects of managed care on prices and how the magnitude of these effects is influenced by the level of competition in hospital markets.[6] Studies conducted using data from periods prior to the mid-1980s generally found results consistent with the existence of a medical arms race or quality competition rather than price competition. Robinson & Luft (1985, 1987) found that the more competitive market structures, those with more hospitals or lower Herfindahl indices, had higher costs, in two studies, one using nationwide hospital data from 1972 and 1973 and one comparing hospital market performance in 1972 with that in 1982.

Robinson & Luft (1988) found quite different results in a study comparing changes in hospital costs from 1982 to 1986 in California with those in the control group of hospitals in 43 states. They found that 'pro competitive or market oriented' policies undertaken in California resulted in 'rates of inflation in average costs per admission 10.1 per cent lower (in California hospitals) than in the control group.' They concluded the pro-competitive policies were 'bearing fruit'. Numerous studies have found evidence that competition results in lower costs, price cost margins and prices. These studies used transaction prices rather than list prices. The latter were used in a number of studies in which it was found that more competition resulted in higher prices (Davis, 1971, and Chirikos, 1989). Dranove et al (1993) calculated price cost margins for a collection of hospital services using transaction prices for hospitals in California for 1983 and 1988. They found no relationship between price cost margins in 1983 but found that increases in competition (as reflected in reductions in the Herfindahl index) resulted in lower price cost margins in 1988. Gruber (1992) confirmed this result for California hospitals using different statistical procedures. Dranove & White (1994) conclude this evidence supports the hypothesis that growth in selective contracting increased the sensitivity of price cost margins and transaction prices to the level of competition.

Staten et al (1988) found the Indiana Blue Cross plan received greater discounts in markets with multiple hospitals. Melnick et al (1992) and Zwanziger & Melnick (1988, 1993) reported substantial evidence that competition is impacting hospital costs and prices. Using California data they reported that the cost per admission was higher in markets with more competition in the early 1980s but that the relationship turned around in the mid-1980s. They found the change to be related to competitive pressures on the hospital, such as the existence of multiple providers in the market, the adoption of the Medicare PPS, and the growth of managed care. Thus, they concluded that competition had greatly reduced and possibly eliminated the medical arms race.

In another study Melnick et al (1992) examined the impact of competition on price by comparing the relationship between final prices negotiated by Blue Cross of California and hospital competition. They found negotiated prices to be lower in markets with more hospitals.[7] The results generated by the turnaround in the form of competition that began in the early 1980s are quite strong and clear: prices and costs are lower in competitive hospital markets. Let us emphasize our reason for laboriously providing this evidence. The lower prices under competition occurred because states passed enabling legislation to permit HMOs and PPOs to steer patients to more efficient providers.[8]

8.4 EVIDENCE FROM THE STATE OF WASHINGTON

In this section we provide empirical estimates, derived from an earlier study by Arnould et al (1995), of the benefits from increased competition. That study considered the effects of antitrust immunity in the state of Washington. The methodology involved using different methods to estimate the benefits of competition, including the percentage of the population living in markets served by multiple providers as well as use of estimates produced by previously published research.

8.4.1 Impact of competition: evidence from studies of other states

Earlier we reported a study by Melnick et al (1992) that investigated the effect of competition in hospital markets in California on the price paid by a managed-care insurance firm that negotiated preferred provider rates for its enrollees. Specifically, their measure of price was the actual average price per day net of discounts paid for in-patient care by Blue Cross of California in 1987. They used multiple regression techniques to account for other differences in the demographic characteristics of the market, as well as case-mix characteristics of the hospital. Finally, they used a weighted Herfindahl index to develop a hospital-specific (rather than the traditional antitrust-market-specific) measure of the degree of competition the hospital faced from other hospitals.[9] Regressing these variables on the prices Blue Cross negotiated with hospitals, they found the following specific results measuring the impact of competition on hospital rates:

- hospitals in more competitive markets (those having lower Herfindahl indices) also charged lower prices to Blue Cross. After adjusting for other factors mentioned above, the authors found that markets with three equally-sized hospitals charged prices that, on average, were 9 per cent lower than the prices charged by hospitals in markets with two equally-sized hospitals. A decrease in the number of equally-sized hospitals in the market from four to three resulted in a price increase of about 4.7 per cent on average. Finally, markets with two equally-sized competitors charged prices to Blue Cross that were 17.1 per cent less on average than those charged by hospitals in single hospital markets;[10]

- Blue Cross was able to negotiate lower prices when their enrollees accounted for a larger proportion of a hospital's total patient days – in other words, in cases where the hospital was more dependent upon Blue Cross for business;
- Blue Cross had to pay higher prices to hospitals when those hospitals accounted for a larger share of Blue Cross's patient days within the hospital's market. This effect was intensified in markets that were more concentrated.

This analysis controlled for cost differences among the hospitals. The authors found that lowering costs would lower prices, too. However, they estimated that it would require a 24 per cent decline in costs to counteract the 9 per cent increase in price brought about by a decline in the number of hospitals from three to two. Even more dramatic, costs would have to decline by over 46 per cent to counteract the 17.1 per cent increase in price brought about by a drop from a two to one hospital market.

The magnitudes of the effects of competition estimated in the Melnick et al (1992) study have been chosen from among the many studies discussed earlier, because, unlike most other studies Melnick et al (1992) provide a direct comparison of the impact of competition on the prices paid by a managed-care insurer. Also, this study is widely considered to be one of the most thorough and carefully conducted analyses of these effects. However, we believe the true importance of this benchmark is that it provides evidence of the substantial magnitude of the benefits derived from competition

in the form of lower prices. Therefore it provides a measure of the gains that must be forthcoming from situations in which antitrust immunity might be granted if those situations permit a decline in the number of effective competitors (in this case, hospitals) in health-care markets.

8.4.2 Impact of competition: evidence from analyses of Washington markets

We turn now to an analysis of the impact of competition in hospital markets in Washington using data that describe these hospitals and markets. Essentially, this approach attempted to reproduce the Melnick et al (1992) study as closely as possible using data from Washington markets. This path was important for two reasons. First, as mentioned above, the Melnick et al procedure has been widely praised as a sound research methodology. Second, since the Arnould et al (1995) results are statistically similar to the Melnick et al results, we have evidence of the robust nature of the procedure and the results. In addition, this gives us more confidence to make inferences from some of the Melnick et al results on data not available in the Arnould et al (1995) study of the State of Washington.

Two sources of data were used to analyse the impact of competition on Washington markets. First, financial data were provided for all hospitals in Washington by the Washington Department of Health. Patient-origin data used to delineate markets and determine the share of managed care in each hospital were taken from the Washington Department of Health's Comprehensive Hospital Abstract Reporting System (CHARS) data. Demographic data were taken from the Area Resource File prepared by the US Department of Health and Human Services (HHS). Limited data were provided, on a confidential basis, by some of the HMOs and PPOs which operate in the state of Washington. In limited instances these provided direct measures of the prices and contract conditions negotiated by these managed-care providers.

Results using hospital average-revenue data

Multiple regression techniques similar to those used by Melnick et al were employed using data specific to Washington hospitals to estimate the impact of competition on average hospital daily revenue in Washington. Specifically, a coefficient was estimated that indicates how much an increase in the level of the measure of competition will change average daily revenue – the dependent variable – holding other factors or variables in the estimated equation at their mean values.

Appropriate measures of price and competition were identified to determine the influence of changes in the level of competition on price. The data identified charges by hospital, broken down along several patient categories, for all hospitals in the state. However, charges are not the best measure of prices because many payers are granted various levels of discounts. However, the information on discounts necessary to calculate actual hospital revenue was not available.

Data also are available from the Department of Health's financial data set that identify actual revenue. Revenues and patient days are provided for Medicaid, Medicare, and 'other' patients. The last category includes mostly private-pay patients. The Department of Health also provided cost data across all categories for each hospital, both with and without adjustments (for items such as recoveries). From these data, average revenue per patient day was computed as was average cost per patient day.

One problem with these measures of average cost and revenue is that they could be influenced by the mix of DRGs treated by the hospital. One of the powers of multiple regression is to account for the influence of other factors such as case-mix. Other variables were included in the estimations that are intended to account for the influence of differences in the mix of DRGs.

Two measures of competition were used. The first was the HHI used by Melnick et al (1992). This variable has larger values with higher levels in concentration (i.e. reductions in competition). The second measure of competition was a raw count of the number of hospitals in the market,

where markets are defined using the rules outlined in Dranove et al (1992). They defined the market as including all hospitals within 10 miles of one another or within an urban area, if the hospital in question was located in an urban area. If all hospitals in a market were of equal size, the two measures of competition would be perfectly correlated. In fact the size distribution of hospitals in multiple hospital markets was so uneven that the correlation between these variables was not extremely high.

It is important to identify variables that measure differences between the hospitals that might cause differences in per-day prices. There are differences other than the level of competition in the markets in which they are located. First, following the lead of Melnick et al (1992), a hospital-specific cost index is included. Hospitals with higher costs are expected to charge higher prices holding the level of competition constant. This is especially so if the higher costs are the result of higher quality, more complex cases or other differences in the mix of DRGs treated by the hospital.

Strong evidence was found of the beneficial impact of competition on hospital prices. Significantly, the results of estimates using data for hospitals in Washington were surprisingly consistent with the results of Melnick et al (1992). The estimated coefficient that measures the impact of changes in the HHI (competition) on prices was highly significant. The results in an analysis that included only the effect of changes in the HHI indicate that a change from three equally-sized competing hospitals to two would be expected to increase prices by about 23 per cent; dropping from two to one would increase prices an additional 39 per cent. If the second measure of competition is included, the shift from three hospitals to two would increase prices 26 per cent and the reduction from two to one would increase prices 43.6 per cent. These estimates are slightly greater in magnitude than comparable estimates by Melnick et al (1992), which may be due to the fact that managed-care systems generally are larger and account for a larger share of the market in California than in Washington.

Turning to the focus of the present essay, it is important to control for the impact of the degree to which the hospital was reliant upon managed-care plans for revenue. The data for total hospital charges by payer type were available for all hospitals in Washington from a special report developed by the Department of Health using data contained in the patient discharge reports. The percentage of total charges to HMOs and PPOs (contract insurers) was used to measure the penetration of managed-care plans into hospitals' businesses. The coefficient for this variable had the expected negative sign, indicating that as the proportion of business accounted for by HMO/PPO increases for any hospital, the price per non-Medicare/non-Medicaid patient decreases. The size of the coefficient was remarkably close in magnitude to the estimate of Melnick et al (1992), even though the Washington-State coefficient was not statistically significant at an acceptable level of confidence. The lack of statistical precision may be due to the fact that data required use of gross charges rather than net revenues received after discounts and allowances. Since hospital charges frequently differ from actual receipts, using charge data introduces an element of variation that could weaken the apparent strength of the relationship between prices and managed-care penetration.

In summary, Arnould et al (1995) demonstrated that the types of benefits derived from competition in the form of lower charges in other states have been replicated in Washington hospitals. Using the Washington-specific results provides even stronger estimates of these benefits. This is a measure of the potential for greater losses if antitrust immunity is used to permit reduction in the level of competition in hospital markets. This is particularly true for those hospital markets with a small number of providers. Any loss in the degree of competition would have to be offset by significant efficiency increases, but immunity would not be required in such cases.

8.5 MARKET STRUCTURE AND THE HOSPITAL INDUSTRY

We have discussed competitive reforms; how they began and how they have affected several aspects of the healthcare industry. Now we will

take a closer look at the hospital industry and some of the changes in market structure, specifically horizontal mergers and acquisitions, which have taken place during the time leading up to and during competitive reform. We will outline two merger waves, one of which occurred in the 1970s and early 1980s, and was a result of incentives provided by the Medicare and Medicaid reimbursement and capital investment incentives and the second wave occurred in the early 1990s. While this first merger wave was not a result of managed care, it is still important here for two reasons. First, it was during this time that investor-owned hospitals appeared in the market and the first large systems began developing and expanding. In addition, most of the empirical work which has been done on hospital mergers utilises data from the first merger wave.

Incentives among providers to engage in various types of horizontal and vertical integration stem from four general factors related to the increase in competition in healthcare markets. First, excess capacity and declining margins have led to horizontal and vertical integration to achieve production economies, consolidate operations and reduce inefficient duplication of services. Mergers and looser affiliations have occurred among hospitals in different geographic markets across the US to gain efficiencies from participating in large purchasing co-operatives and to gain preferred access to capital markets.

Second, providers have engaged in various degrees of horizontal and vertical integration to reduce transactions or contracting costs. Transactions costs result from (1) the volume of contracts required; (2) the inability to clearly stipulate some element of the service to be delivered, such as quality; and (3) asset specificity, i.e. the need to invest in assets that might last beyond the length of the contract but have no alternative uses (Williamson, 1985). In most managed-care situations, contracts are required between managed-care firms and a large number of providers, including physicians, hospitals and other types of providers. The volume of independent contracts is reduced by physicians who practice independently and participate in Independent Practice

Arrangements (IPAs), which have the responsibility of contracting with HMOs and PPOs for these physicians. Similarly, physician group-practices have grown rapidly to reduce transactions costs. Hospitals in single markets have merged to provide more geographic choice to a managed-care organisation. Hos- pitals have integrated with skilled nursing facilities, home care units and other types of provider to have a more complete service offering and to be able to provide the most efficient level of service for its patients. Often, this is accomplished by merger, owing to the difficulty of specifying all desired conditions for service delivery in a contract. Finally, joint ventures may be required to provide for the appropriate level of utilisation of costly technology. Hos- pitals have contracted with physicians (PHOs) to assure a flow of patients to the hospital.

Third, providers often integrate to attain a scale of operation consistent with the level of risk-bearing the organisation must absorb. Risk may result from the desire on the part of a managed-care firm to capitate providers. Clearly, a minimum size is necessary for providers to undertake this level of risk. In numerous situations in the US, providers have taken on substantial risk by integrating directly into the insurance market. Many hospitals and large physician groups offer risk-bearing managed-care (insurance) products. There is substantial evidence of minimal optimal scale of operation of these managed-care insurers. Scale spreads administrative costs across more members and also improves the predictability of outcomes.

Fourth, horizontal and vertical integration may occur for the purpose of increasing monopoly power and reducing competitive outcomes of competitive reforms and managed-care products. Actions against a number of mergers and other contractual arrangements by the enforcers of the antitrust laws in the US have become common.

The degree of integration is defined by the volume and diversity of units brought together. It is also defined along the dimensions of the tightness and completeness of the contract. Integration may be within the confines of horizontal markets or across horizontally and vertically related·markets. Degrees of integration also may vary from loose contracting to complete mergers (Nichols, 1996). Keeping these factors in mind, we will now examine the trends in hospital mergers and consolidations starting in the 1970s.

8.5.1 Early government programmes

At the same time as insurance coverage in the US was expanding due to employer benefit programmes and new tax laws, Congress was also passing legislation aimed at expanding and upgrading hospitals. The Hill–Burton Act of 1945 was enacted to provide federal funds, along with state and local matching funds, for building new hospital structures or providing upgrades and repair to existing buildings. During this time, there were few hospital closures or consolidations as the Hill–Burton Act provided the assistance necessary to keep many poorly performing hospitals in business.

When the US federal government passed Medicare and Medicaid into law in 1965, the incentive structure for the hospital industry changed. These programmes were a compromise between those favouring a more comprehensive national healthcare programme and the strong medical organisations, which feared Government involvement in the industry. In the compromise, providers were able to protect their interests by mandating provisions which maintained autonomy in medical decisions and pricing. In addition, the new law contained provisions which reimbursed hospitals for a reasonable rate of return on equity capital and allowed depreciation to be computed on the basis of replacement cost as opposed to historical cost. The Government had agreed to write physicians and hospitals a blank cheque for the care of eligible participants and it provided cash for capital expansion by hospitals.

There were no incentives for hospitals to cut costs and there were incentives for capital expenditures, which helped to encourage the medical arms race. Not surprisingly, hospitals during this time earned unusually large profits. Hospitals were interested in taking advantage of these benefits; growth of facilities, both by the acquisition of new hospitals and expansion of existing facilities, translated into higher profits. As Hoy & Gray (1986) point out, the easiest way for hospitals to reap the benefits from quick growth is to merge with facilities already in existence. This incentive structure had two effects. It led to the growth of investor-owned hospitals and to an increase in the number and size of hospital systems. The latter was accomplished through an increase in the number of mergers and acquisitions in the hospital industry.

8.5.2 The emergence of investor-owned hospitals and growth of multihospital systems

For-profit hospitals were in existence long before the Medicare and Medicaid programmes started. Yet it was not until after Medicare and Medicaid began that a new type of for-profit institution, investor-owned hospitals, began to emerge. An investor-owned hospital, hereafter IO hospital, differs from other proprietary institutions in ownership and size. IO hospitals are owned mostly by shareholders and are usually part of an IO system which owns and operates several facilities.

In 1975 there were 378 IO hospitals in the US containing 51,230 beds. This jumped dramatically to 878 hospitals and 113,122 beds in 1984. Similarly, the percentage of total hospitals which were IO also doubled, moving from 6.3 per cent in 1975 to 13.1 per cent in 1983 (Gray, 1986). And as stated above, many of these IO hospitals were a part of a multihospital system.[11] From 1977 to 1983 the number of IO systems increased at an average annual rate of 10.3 per cent. The number of hospitals per system was also increasing at an average annual rate of 7.9 per cent, and at the same time, the number of independent IO hospitals was declining (Ermann & Gabel, 1986). Non-profit hospital systems were also growing over the same time period; however Ermann & Gabel (1984) determined their growth rate to be slower than that of IO systems, with an average rate of 3.5 per cent from 1978 to 1982. In summary, there are two changes taking place in the industry over this time period. First, IO hospitals were increasing in number and there was also large growth in the number of hospital systems in the US, many of which were IO systems.

We have already discussed the first reason for the expansion and merging of hospital groups in the late 1970s and early 1980s. There were excess profits being made and incentives for capital expansion. In order to take advantage of the available profits, the hospital groups choose the fastest avenue for growth, acquisition.[12] Hoy & Gray (1986) conducted a study in 1984 of the six largest IO hospital systems in the US.[13] Through 1984 there were 540 hospitals acquired by these six conglomerates. Of these 540 'new' IO system hospitals, only 20 per cent were constructed by the parent IO system. Purchased hospitals comprised 68 per cent of the total while 12 per cent were acquired through leasing arrangements by the controlling company. These new organisations were growing because of the incentive structures, which induced system development, and for other reasons.

Ermann & Gabel (1984, 1986) offer an explanation for the rapid growth of the larger organisations by outlining three advantages multihospital systems have over independently owned hospitals. First, multihospital groups can take advantage of economic benefits which include greater access to capital and economies of scale.[14] Secondly, there are personnel and management benefits for larger systems. Larger companies will be better able to recruit and train workers, which enables them to maintain a higher quality staff. Finally, there are similar planning, programme, and organisational benefits to having several hospitals involved in a system. These advantages, coupled with the new federal programmes and capital investment incentives, led to the huge increases in the number of both IO hospitals and multihospital systems.

Interestingly, despite the advantages of multihospital systems given by Ermann & Gabel (1984, 1986), 18 empirical studies reviewed by Ermann & Gabel (1984) concluded that systems of hospitals have higher costs than independent hospitals.[15] Additionally, studies conducted in the 1980s examining the differences between independent and systems hospitals found no differences in quality of care, access, or service for the poor. Morrisey & Alexander (1987) point to two flaws in these studies which may have caused the unpredictable results. First, the studies rely on the implicit assumption that hospitals are randomly selected into a system. There is no reason to believe this would be true and it seems more likely that hospitals in systems have some specific characteristics which differ from those of hospitals which have not joined a system. Second, these studies have not taken into consideration the possibility that there are differences between systems and their hospitals. For example, the differentiating characteristic leading to these results may be their type of ownership (for-profit, IO, non-profit, etc.) instead of system ownership.[16]

8.5.3 Multihospital systems and competitive reforms

The wave of mergers and system growth in the late 1970s and early 1980s did not continue. As detailed earlier, this was the time period which saw the onset of competitive reforms, and they impacted upon the expansion in the industry. Reardon & Reardon (1995) offer two explanations for the end of the expansion period: 1) the federal government decreased depreciation payments to hospitals and began to watch the payment activities of merging hospitals more closely (i.e., CON legislation); and 2) the federal government eliminated the existing Medicare cost-reimbursement programme and began the DRG system, allowing hospitals to keep any reimbursement greater than actual costs, which provided the hospitals with incentives to cut costs. The retrospective fee for service payment system was no longer in effect and the opportunity for excess profits seemed to be gone. 'As a result, the large IO hospital systems were forced to retrench and divest.'[17]

The slowdown in IO system growth caused by the new emphasis on cost containment did not mean the end of system growth. The new cost-containment strategies led to increased uncertainty and concern about profitability. Excess capacity needed to be decreased and hospitals were having difficulty adjusting to the new type of incentive put forth by the federal government. This led to a number of different kinds of structural change, one of which was a resurgence of horizontal integration (Watt et al, 1986, Reardon & Reardon, 1995). Therefore, the cost containment which initially slowed consolidation in the hospital industry by trying to eliminate excess profits eventually brought more integration for very different reasons. Now hospitals were trying to adapt to the new incentive structure, remain profitable and, in many cases, survive.

8.5.4 The hospital industry in the present day

Consolidation of hospitals and the creation of large hospital conglomerates resumed in the 1990s. Reardon & Reardon (1995) review the current characteristics of the hospital industry focusing specifically on hospital systems. They report that in 1993, seven of the largest ten hospital systems were IO and the remaining three systems were owned by the federal government (military hospital systems and public health services). These ten systems collectively own 15.4 per cent of all hospitals and 14.8 per cent of all beds in the US. The number of hospitals owned by each varies from the largest with 245 to the smallest with 39.

In the same study, Reardon & Reardon (1995) use data from the AHA 1987 and 1992 annual studies to examine hospital system attributes. With the SMSA as the relevant market, they calculated concentration ratios for the 21 largest urban areas in the US in 1987 and 1992.[18] The mean concentration ratio increased from 27.0 in 1987 to 30.5 in 1992 for an increase of 13 per cent. Furthermore, the mean percentage of system-owned hospitals in the 21 urban areas increased 3.6 per cent (from 44.8 per cent in 1987 to 46.4 per cent in 1992) and there was an even larger increase in the mean percentage of system-owned beds (9.6 per cent, in the same 21 areas).

These results suggest that hospital markets are still becoming more concentrated and, more importantly, hospital *systems* are controlling a larger percentage of hospitals. Considering these changes in market structure, we will now look to the question of why these consolidations are taking place and what kind of an impact they will have on the industry as a whole.

8.6 MEASURING THE IMPACT OF HOSPITAL MERGERS

The competitive paradigm teaches that there will be many buyers and many sellers, none of whom have enough market power to affect prices or quantities. Competition will eliminate any excess profits through arbitrage and the market will always move to the equilibrium price and quantity. Unfortunately, few markets follow this paradigm and, as explained earlier, the healthcare industry has severe informational asymmetries and uncertainty problems which inhibit the competitive market's efficient outcome. This complicates the analysis considerably.

Increases in hospital mergers and, therefore, increases in market concentration could have two basic effects. On one hand, the increase in market concentration may create economies of scale or economies of scope bringing about decreases in production costs for the hospital, which will raise the equilibrium level of output. Alternatively, the increase in market concentration may give the hospital considerable bargaining power with insurers making it possible for them to demand higher prices for the same products. All hospitals in the market would be able to restrict output and raise prices. These two effects clearly work against one another, and it is difficult to learn which will prevail in any given circumstance. In addition, there are also issues of access and quality which may be affected by changes in market structure.[19]

8.6.1 Market power vs efficiency

Woolley (1989) conducted an event study aimed at measuring the competitive impact of hospital mergers. His results, along with the comment by Vita & Schumann (1991) also address the question of why these mergers are occurring. Woolley (1989) uses 29 different events taking place from 1969 to 1985 among large hospital systems, which he labels as pro-merger (i.e. a merger announcement) or anti-merger (i.e. filing of an antitrust suit). Using the traditional event-study method, Woolley (1989) measures stock value prices for rival firms during an event window around the time of the pro-merger or anti-merger event.[20] He finds that pro-merger events had a positive effect on the market value of rival firms and anti-merger events had a negative effect on the market value of rival firms. This finding is consistent with traditional oligopoly theory which argues that mergers increase market concentration making it possible for all firms in the market to earn supracompetitive profits. In other words, the change in market power for all firms resulting from the merger overrides any cost reductions which may result from efficiencies.

Vita & Schumann (1991) provide a criticism of Woolley's findings arguing that 1) Woolley (1989) used events which were not horizontal transactions; 2) the change in concentration was too small to make a difference; or 3) the firms were not rivals and, therefore, the abnormal returns could not have been caused by the merger event. Vita & Schumann (1991) examined 15 of his events case by case attempting to show that all contained one of the three problems described above. They use this analysis to change Woolley's proposition about the reason for hospital mergers.

Vita & Schumann (1991) assert that because Woolley (1989) is wrong, the market power rationale of mergers cannot be supported. Furthermore, there were abnormal returns for these firms, which were not rivals, during the event window, and these must have been caused by something other than the merger event. Their theory is that the abnormal returns, in fact, were caused by information about efficiencies being revealed by the merger event. In other words, when two firms announce a merger, this provides other similar hospitals with information concerning efficiencies which will make them more profitable thereby increasing their firm value. This theory supports the efficiency rationale for mergers.

Woolley (1991) defends his earlier work by making two major points in the face of the criticism. First, Woolley argues that Vita & Schumann (1991) are working with incomplete information. They formed their markets by county without regard to neighbouring hospitals in different counties therefore missing several rivals. They also failed to take into account competitors who were competing with firms in markets other than the one where the announcement took place.[21] Second, Woolley (1991) argues that any informational benefit which would arise from a merger event would be available to all firms. Therefore, any cost efficiencies would be exploited by all firms, leaving profits unchanged.

8.6.2 Ownership and the market vs efficiency question

The Department of Justice has taken the stance that all hospitals, regardless of ownership, will face the same standard in the application of antitrust law on the understanding that non-profit firms will take advantage of market power to increase prices, and therefore profits, in a manner similar to for-profit firms. In an effort to examine the appropriateness of this standard, Lynk (1995a) applies the market power versus efficiency question to non-profit hospitals by evaluating a model comparing the behaviour of for-profit and non-profit hospitals.[22]

Lynk's model tests the behaviour of hospital prices, as a function of market concentration and market share, before and after a merger. Hospitals are characterised as non-profit, for-profit, and public. Lynk (1995a) finds the merger effects do vary by ownership. A merger of two for-profit hospitals, each with 25 per cent market share, is associated with a 5.8 per cent increase in prices. A merger of two non-profit hospitals, each with 25 per cent market share, is associated with a price decrease of 4.1 per cent, but a merger of two public facilities, each with 25 per cent market share is associated with a 5.1 per cent increase in prices. The distinction between non-profit and public hospitals is important here. Contrary to intuition, Government-owned non-profit hospitals behave very differently from their private non-profit counterparts.

These results suggest that for-profit hospitals and non-profit hospitals do not act similarly: for-profit hospitals seem to be reaping the benefits of increased market power while non-profit hospitals are taking advantage of cost efficiencies resulting from the merger. At first glance, the public hospital result seems odd. However, all through the empirical results, the public hospital behaves more like a for-profit institution. Lynk's explanation turns to the hospital's treatment of excess profits. For-profit institutions distribute excess profits to the owners, whether they be shareholders or private individuals, as dividends and capital gains. Non-profit hospitals presumably have differing objectives. Consider a community-run non-profit hospital which acts something like a co-operative. Cost savings and profits are most likely turned back to the organisation. Government-owned non-profit hospitals, on the other hand, have different incentives. Excess profits can be used in other areas of the Government (i.e. building new roads, improving education, etc.) thereby giving the Government the same incentive structure as the for-profit firm.

If for-profit and non-profit institutions do act differently, as the results suggest, the Department of Justice should consider ownership status when determining whether a hospital is in violation of antitrust law. While it is clear that the law should prevent hospitals from merging for the purposes of gaining market power in order to earn supracompetitive prices, it is hard to justify enforcing the same standard on a community group merging for the purposes of providing medical care to their own community in the most cost-effective manner.

8.6.3 The impact of mergers on hospital costs

Another estimate of the effect of hospital consolidation is found in the literature on hospital cost functions and economies of scale and scope in hospital production. If increases in firm size bring about decreases in average cost, then there are economies of scale, and hospital mergers among hospitals in the production range of decreasing average costs would bring about decreases in the cost of care. Similarly, economies of scope occur when decreases in average cost are realised by producing different services; taking advantage of resources which can be used for the joint production of multiple products.

The literature on economics of scale and scope is discussed in Chapter 6, but it appears clear that there is no compelling expectation of significant efficiency gains from merger. The hospital organisation is extremely complex, making it difficult for researchers to explicitly model and estimate costs of firms in the industry. In addition to these modelling problems, no two mergers are alike. They vary from total merger, where two departments are combined into one, to the opposite extreme where both facilities continue operating as if there had been no change of ownership. The impacts of mergers then will vary as much as the type of merger.

Clearly, the policy impacts of changes in any of the preceding market characteristics are very important. There are implications for the regulating authorities and courts which are now beginning to confront antitrust cases for merging hospitals. The manner in which the authorities rule on the legality of hospital mergers is important and requires careful consideration of the impact of mergers on efficiency and market power. Obviously managed care generates incentives for increased efficiency by being able to move patients from one provider to another, but increased efficiency, to the extent it is dependent upon hospital consolidations, reduces the options available to managed-care organisations.

8.7 ISSUES SURROUNDING ANTITRUST ENFORCEMENT

The growth of managed-care programmes has been very directly aided by antitrust intervention, as documented in earlier sections of this chapter. With the recent changes in the structure of the hospital industry, antitrust issues have remained in the forefront. Regulatory agencies have examined the issues trying to determine the appropriate standards for application in cases of integration in the healthcare market.

The underlying structures of the managed-care programmes vary dramatically across

plans. These differences are usually in the forms of contracts between the insurer and the providers. These contracts have much divergence both across and within plans. These differences have brought about claims, usually by provider groups, that their inability to collectively establish prices charged for their services to managed-care programmes without risk of violation of antitrust laws has led to inefficiencies and an uneven playing field.

In 1992, the Department of Justice (DOJ) and the Federal Trade Commission (FTC) issued *Horizontal Merger Guidelines* which set out the standards to be used in cases of provider integration. This report summarized the standards under five headings: 1) market concentration, 2) possible adverse competitive effects, 3) ease of market entry, 4) efficiencies gained and 5) the possibility of the providers' failure in absence of merger.[23] The basic standard, when looking at these five areas, is to determine if the merger will, overall, have positive or negative effects on the market in question. All mergers will result in gains and losses, the only problem is to determine which will dominate in the given situation.

In this section, we describe areas in which antitrust litigation might be applied and describe the potential gains and losses from antitrust immunity in each case. The material here is concerned more with the economic issues. Interested readers should see Flynn (1994) for a more detailed discussion of the case history in this area.

8.7.1 Horizontal actions

Horizontal actions generally take three forms among hospitals, physicians and other providers: mergers, joint ventures and loose net agreements.[24] In all cases the economic question is whether the actions enhance efficiency or merely increase market power. The latter is particularly troublesome if the market power is sufficient to substantially lessen competition or reaches the point of giving the unit monopoly power or the ability to function as a cartel. Mergers of horizontal competitors increase market power by eliminating a competitor. Mergers between hospitals may significantly increase market power in hospital markets with small numbers of hospitals or in markets in which one of the parties to the merger was a significant competitor.

Managed-care plans have brought about a significant reduction in hospital admissions, and average lengths of stay for those admitted, and a movement to either one-day surgeries or out-patient surgeries, some of which are no longer conducted at hospitals.[25] Some hospitals with excess capacity have turned to mergers with other hospitals, often in the same market. If these hospitals account for a substantial share of the market, the merger may increase market power to the extent that it represents a substantial lessening of competition. The merger could threaten competition by reducing the alternative sources of supply to managed-care firms, thereby reducing price and quality competition. The reduction in price competition brought about by the merger may be particularly harmful in hospital markets because many hospital markets are tight oligopolists.[26]

It is commonly argued that it would be more efficient in areas plagued with excess capacity to permit the hospitals to jointly determine and allocate the services to be offered by each hospital. However, mergers in which substantial, measurable gains in efficiency result from consolidation of operations are not prohibited under current antitrust guidelines and enforcement policies. This is also true when one or both of the merging parties is likely to fail without the merger, or when the change in market structure is not substantial. Similarly, hospitals are permitted to 'spin-off' activities into joint ventures when gains in efficiency can be documented along with demand that is inadequate to support multiple providers.

Horizontal actions among physicians involve mergers of practices much as in the case of hospitals. Alternatively, the horizontal action could be the formation of joint ventures and other arrangements through which the physicians form networks to negotiate with managed-care firms. These include such entities as IPAs, PPOs, and group and staff model HMOs. The alleged benefits of the organisations are increased efficiencies and reduced transaction costs in the process of negotiating

managed-care agreements. In networks, whether formed by merger or contractual arrangements, only one transaction is needed to negotiate an agreement with a number of physicians. Additional economies may be achieved through agreement of common management of the network/managed-care firms. Outright horizontal mergers among physicians must be viewed just as were hospital mergers. Gains in market power must be weighed against gains in efficiency.

Co-operative behaviour among physicians in the same market becomes very problematic if it involves collective price setting. Collective action to set prices by networks of physicians in many circumstances constitutes horizontal price fixing. In these situations, the economic result is to reduce competition and raise the price charged to the managed-care providers.

Collective price setting by physician networks may reduce competition in two additional ways. First, there may be a spillover effect from network to non-network activities. Prices set in the network may become prices charged to payers outside the units negotiated by the networks. Second, the size of the network may function as a barrier to entry to the formation of other competitive networks. For example, if the network attracts more physicians than necessary to provide services to a managed-care plan, this excess capacity could have a negative spill-over effect. The network may be capturing so much of the physician-services market that other viable networks are precluded from forming.

8.7.2 Vertical actions

Vertical actions usually involve the formation of some form of integrated delivery system (IDS). Different types of providers are integrated, either through merger and ownership or through contractual arrangements, to provide an integrated set of healthcare services to an insured population. In some instances, the IDS incorporates the insurance function. These include management service organisations (MSOs), physician hospital organisations (PHOs) and foundation integrated delivery systems. However, there are many variations of organisational form and also a varying degree of formality to the relationships among providers contained within each of these general rubrics.

There are multiple potential benefits from the formation of an IDS. As in the case of physician networks just described, transaction costs may be reduced. An IDS may reduce costs by integrating the management of patient treatments. Also, an IDS may provide better mechanisms to evaluate and control the quality of each unit or provider in the network.

There are numerous potential negative effects IDSs could have on competition in healthcare markets. First, the base of economic power in a vertically integrated system is usually horizontal market power in one or more of the markets in which the IDS operates. The IDS may be used to justify mergers or collusive arrangements among physicians beyond the level necessary to achieve efficiency of operation of the IDS.

Of particular concern in many healthcare markets is the fact that many of them are served by three or fewer hospitals. Suppose the market was served by one hospital. Physicians and other providers could organise around the single hospital, for example, using the hospital as a cartel manager. This would not change the competitive outcome in the already monopolised hospital segment of the market but it could significantly reduce competition in the physician segment of the market; normally, it is quite possible that the physician submarket could function with some degree of competitiveness. The direct economic effect of this reduction in competition may be to reduce competition in the physician-services market bringing about increased physician charges or a reduced willingness on the part of physicians to negotiate competitive contracts. It also will increase the price of managed-care contracts in this market by prohibiting or restricting entry of other managed-care plans. If alternative plans do enter the market presumably they all will face higher prices. The hospital thus functions in the role Krattenmacher & Salop (1986) refer to as the cartel ringmaster.

A second way in which vertical integration of the type being undertaken by IDSs could potentially reduce competition in some or all health-services markets may come about if the segment of the market left outside the IDS is very concentrated. For example, suppose there are two hospitals in the market and one forms an IDS that contains a managed-care insurance programme. If the IDS exclusively provides services through its self-contained insurance plan, other potential entrants into the managed-care insurance market are left with a single hospital with which to negotiate a managed-care agreement. Under various circumstances this single remaining hospital may have the ability to charge the potential entrant a 'monopoly price'. In effect the IDS may be able to impede entry or control the level of competition by raising the rival's costs in a very direct manner. This may also be accomplished in an indirect manner by the impact the actions of the IDS have on the structure of the remaining segment of the market.

8.8 CONCLUSION

The healthcare industry in the US has changed dramatically in the last 30 years. Managed care changed the incentive structure, encouraging efficiency in a market which had not previously competed on the basis of price. Providers were no longer encouraged to improve the quality of the healthcare product through the medical arms race, but were instead encouraged to cut costs. The new incentives have affected all areas of healthcare provision, including the structure of the hospital industry. We have summarised some of those changes and effects here to provide a framework for understanding the US experience.

We began by considering the impetus for changes in the healthcare sector. We provided an overview of the competitive reforms which have brought about change in the structure of incentives. We then outlined the expected benefit of competitive reforms, namely managed care, looking more closely at the changes in hospital competition. Our survey of the evidence shows that increases in competition *do* lower the prices of medical care in both the hospital and physician markets. Specific studies in California and Washington hospital markets reveal that decreases in price are associated with increases in the number of hospitals in a market. The magnitude of this effect is somewhat reduced by an offsetting increase in costs resulting from losses of efficiency, also due to the increase in the number of hospitals in a market.

Of particular interest to this chapter is the experience of the US hospital industry. We examined the changes in market structure which have taken place. One major change is the significant consolidation observed in provider markets, specifically the hospital industry. Providers will consolidate for one of two reasons; to become more efficient or to gain market power. The first will lower costs of production for the provider, and this should be reflected in lower prices for the consumer. The latter will allow the provider to raise prices for the consumer by taking advantage of the lack of alternatives for those seeking healthcare. While there is a wealth of knowledge concerning these two trade-offs in the hospital industry in theory, it is difficult to explicitly measure the results due to the difficulty in modelling the hospital organisation. The results of studies on these issues have been mixed. There may be efficiencies associated with consolidation in the form of lower costs. However, there is also evidence of higher prices resulting from market power. Our overview ended with the exploration of antitrust considerations. Included in this look at Government intervention was a discussion of the issues surrounding consolidation for regulatory agencies and the courts.

It is hard to overstate the impact that the new competitive healthcare vehicles are having on the contemporary US healthcare sector. As vigorous as it is today, competition in the hospital industry will certainly be an even more important issue in the coming years. Many of the effects of recent mergers and consolidations will take time to surface. In time, as more data become available, many of the studies outlined here will provide the basis for further exploration into the effects of integration. Furthermore, there are even more complex issues, about the effects of vertical integration, which need to be explored.

REFERENCES

Arnould Richard J, DeBrock Lawrence 1995 Physician Compensation as a Strategic Weapon: Competition among HMOs. Manuscript.

Arnould Richard, DeBrock Lawrence, Gift Tom 1995 An Assessment of the Benefits and Costs of Antitrust Immunity for Health Care Providers: Conceptual Models and Empirical Estimates. Report presented to the Attorney General's Office, Washington State, 1995.

Arnould Richard J, Rich Robert F, White William D 1993a Competitive Reforms: Context and Scope. In: Arnould R J, Rich R F, White W D, eds, Competitive Approaches to Health Care Reform, The Urban Institute Press, Washington DC.

Arnould Richard J, Rich Robert F, White William D, Copeland Craig 1993b The Role of Managed Care in Competitive Policy Reforms. In: Arnould R J, Rich R F, White W D, eds, Competitive Approaches to Health Care Reform, The Urban Institute Press, Washington DC.

Bazzoli Gloria J, Marx David Jr, Arnould Richard J, Manheim Larry M 1995 Federal Antitrust Merger Enforcement Standards: A Good Fit for the Hospital industry? Journal of Health Politics, Policy and Law 20:137–169.

Brown Kathryn J, Klosterman Richard E 1986 Hospital Acquisitions and their Effects: Florida, 1979–1982. In: Gray B H, ed. 1986 For-Profit Enterprise in Health Care. National Academy Press, Washington DC.

Chirikos T 1989 Market Competition and Hospital Costs in Florida, 1982–1988. Final report prepared for Florida Health Care Cost Containment Board.

Christensen J B, Sanchez S M, Wholey D R, Shadle M 1991 The HMO Industry: Evolution in Population Demographics and Market Structures. Medical Care Review 48:3–46.

Cowing T G, Holtman A G, Powers S 1983 Hospital Cost Analysis: A Survey and Evaluation of Recent Studies. In: Scheffler R, ed., Advances in Health Economics and Health Services Research, Vol. 4. JAI Press, Greenwich, Ct.

Davis K 1971 Relationship of Hospital Prices to Costs. Applied Economics 4:115–125.

DeBrock Lawrence M, Arnould R J 1992 Utilization Control in HMOs. Quarterly Review of Economics and Finance 32:31–53.

Dranove David, White W D 1994 Recent Theory and Evidence on Competition in Hospital Markets. Journal of Economics & Management Strategy 3:169–209.

Dranove David 1993 The Case for Competitive Reform in Healthcare. In: Arnould R J, Rich R F, White W D, eds, Competitive Approaches to Health Care Reform, The Urban Institute Press, Washington DC.

Dranove David, Shanley M, White W 1993 Price and Concentration in Local Hospital Markets: The Switch from Patient-Driven to Payer-Driven Competition. Journal of Law and Economics 36:179–204.

Dranove David, Shanley M, Simon C 1992 Is Hospital Competition Wasteful? RAND Journal of Economics 23:247–262.

Eliasberg Edward D, 1995 Concerted Healthcare Buying Activities and Antitrust. Utah Law Review pp457–464.

Ermann Dan, Gabel Jon 1986 Investor-Owned Multihospital Systems: A Synthesis of Research Findings. In: Gray B H, ed. For-Profit Enterprise in Health Care. National Academy Press, Washington DC.

Ermann Dan, Gabel Jon 1984 Mulithospital Systems: Issues and Empirical Findings. Health Affairs 3:50–64.

Flynn John J 1994 Antitrust Policy and Health Care Reform. The Antitrust Bulletin, Spring 1994, pp 59–133.

Gift Tom 1997 Essays on Hospital Care: The Impact of Competition on Hospital Prices and the Effects of Medicare & Medicaid HMOs on Utilization and Quality. Unpublished PhD dissertation, University of Illinois at Urbana-Champaign.

Gold M R, Hurley T, Lake T 1995 Arrangements Between Managed Care Plans and Physicians. Physician Payment Review Commission, Washington DC.

Grannemann Thomas W, Brown Randall S, Pauly Mark V 1986 Estimating Hospital Costs: A Multiple-Output Analysis. Journal of Health Economics 5:107–127.

Gray Bradford H, ed. 1986 For-Profit Enterprise in Health Care. National Academy Press, Washington DC.

Gruber J 1992 The Effect of Price Shopping in Medical Markets: Hospital Responses to PPOs in California. Mimeo, MIT.

Havighurst Clark 1995 Antitrust Issues in the Joint Purchasing of Health Care. Utah Law Review, pp409–450.

Havighurst Clark 1988 The Questionable Cost-Containment Record of Commercial Health Insurers. In: Frech H E ed., Health Care in America. Pacific Research Institute for Public Policy, San Francisco.

Hillman A, Pauly M, Kerstein J J 1989 How Do Financial Incentives Affect Physicians' Clinical Decisions and the Financial Pperformance of HMOs? New England Journal of Medicine 321:86–92.

Hoy E W, Gray B H 1986 Trends in the Growth of Major Investor-Owned Hospital Companies. In: Gray B H, ed. For-Profit Enterprise in Health Care. National Academy Press, Washington DC

Iglehart J K 1994 Physicians and the Growth of Managed Care. New England Journal of Medicine 331:1167–1171.

Joskow Paul L 1981 Controlling Hospital Costs: The Role of Government Regulation. MIT Press, Cambridge, MA.

Krattenmacher T, Salop S 1986 Anticompetitive Exclusion: Raising Rivals' Costs to Achieve Power Over Price. Yale Law Journal 96: 266–296.

Lynk William J 1995a Nonprofit Hospital Mergers and the Exercise of Market Power. Journal of Law and Economics 38:437–461.

Lynk William J 1995b The Creation of Economic Efficiencies in Hospital Mergers. Journal of Health Economics 14:507–530.

Melnick Glenn A, Zwanziger Jack, Bamezai Anil, Pattison Robert 1992 The Effect of Market Structure and Bargaining Position on Hospital Prices. Journal of Health Economics 10:217–233.

Morrisey M A, Alexander J A 1987 Hospital Participation in Multihospital Systems. In: Scheffler R M, Rossiter L F, eds. Advances in Health Economics and Health Services Research, Vol. 7. JAI Press, London.

Mullner R M, Anderson R M 1987 A Descriptive and Financial Ratio Analysis of Merged and Consolidated Hospitals: United States, 1980–1985. In: Scheffler R M, Rossiter L F, eds Advances in Health Economics and Health Services Research, Vol. 7. JAI Press, London.

National Center for Health Services Statistics 1992 Health United States 1991. U.S. Public Health Service, Hyatsville, MO.

Nichols Len M 1996 Characteristics of Emerging Health Services Markets and a New Index of Competition Potential. Working Paper. Urban Institute, Washington D.C.

Pauly Mark 1988 A Primer on Competition in Medical Markets. In: Frech H E ed, Health Care in America. Pacific Research Institute for Public Policy, San Francisco.

Reardon Jack, Reardon Laurie 1995 The Restructuring of the Hospital Services Industry. Journal of Economic Issues 29:1063–1081.

Robinson James C, Luft H S 1988 Competition, Regulations, and Hospital Costs, 1982 to 1986. Journal of the American Medical Association 260:2676–2681.

Robinson James C, Luft H S 1987 Competition and the Cost of Hospital Care, 1872 to 1982. Journal of the American Medical Association 257:3241–3245.

Robinson, James C, Luft H S 1985 The Impact of Hospital Market Structure on Patient Volume, Average Length of Stay, and the Cost of Care. Journal of Health Economics 4:333–356.

Schlesinger M, Bentkover J, Blumenthal D, Custer W, Musacchio R, Willer J 1987 Mulithospital Systems and Access to Health-care. In: Scheffler R M, Rossiter L F, eds, Advances in Health Economics and Health Services Research, Vol. 7. JAI Press, London.

Shortell S M 1988 The Evolution of Hospital Systems: Unfulfilled Promises and Self Fulfilling Prophesies. Medical Care Review 45:177–214.

Shortell S M, Morrison E M, Hughes S L, Friedman B S, Vitek J L 1987 Diversification of Health Care Services: the Effects of Ownership, Environment, and Strategy. In: Scheffler R M, Rossiter L F, eds. Advances in Health Economics and Health Services Research, Vol. 7. JAI Press, London.

Simon Carol, White W, Dranove D 1996 The Impact of Managed Care on Physician Incomes: A State by State Analysis. Institute of Government and Public Affairs Working Paper, University of Illinois.

Sloan F A, Morrisey M A, Valvona J 1987 Capital Markets and the Growth of Multihospital Systems. In: Scheffler R M, Rossiter L F, eds., Advances in Health Economics and Health Services Research, Vol. 7. JAI Press, London.

Staten Michael, Dunkelberg William, Umbeck John 1988 Market Share/Market Power Revisited: A New Test for An Old Theory. Journal of Health Economics 7:73–83.

US Congressional Budget Office 1992 Projections of National Health Care Expenditures Washington DC.

Vita M G, Langenfeld J, Paulter P and Miller L 1991 Economic Analysis in Health Care Antitrust. Journal of Contemporary Health Law and Policy 7:73–115.

Vita M G. and Schumann L 1991 The Competitive Effects of Horizontal Mergers in the Hospital Industry: A Closer Look. Journal of Health Economics. 10:359–372.

Vita M G 1990 Exploring Hospital Production Relationships with Flexible Functional Forms. Journal of Health Economics 9:1–21.

Vitaliano Donald F 1987 On the Estimation of Hospital Cost Functions. Journal of Health Economics 6:305–318.

Watt J Michael, Renn Steven C, Hahn James S, Derzon Robert A, Schramm Carl J 1986 The Effects of Ownership and Multihospital System Membership on Hospital Functional Strategies and Economic Performance. In: Gray B H, ed., For-Profit Enterprise in Health Care. National Academy Press, Washington DC.

Williamson Oliver E 1985 The Economic Institutions of Capitalism. The Free Press, New York.

Woolley J M 1991 The Competitive Effects of Horizontal Mergers in the Hospital Industry: An Even Closer Look. Journal of Health Economics 10:373–378.

Woolley J M 1989 The Competitive Effects of Horizontal Mergers in the Hospital Industry. Journal of Health Economics 8:271–291.

Zwanziger Jack, Melnick G A 1993 Effects of Competition on the Hospital Industry: Evidence from California. In: Arnould R J, Rich R F, White W D, ed., Competitive Approaches to Health Care Reform, The Urban Institute Press, Washington DC.

Zwanziger Jack, Melnick G A 1988 The Effects of Hospital Competition and the Medicare PPS Program on Hospital Cost Behavior in California. Journal of Health Economics 7:301–320.

NOTES

1 In the US, the tradition has not been for physicians to be employed by hospitals. Virtually all types of physicians who admit and treat patients in hospitals are granted limited practice privileges in those hospitals but operate as independent enterprises. Most are members of for-profit enterprises who bill patients separately and independently from the hospital. The only exceptions to this form of organisation is for radiologists, pathologists, and anesthesiologists whose services may be provided under a financial contract with the hospital.

2 Pauly (1988) argues that cost containment has public-goods characteristics, thereby eliminating incentives for individual insurers initiatives.

3 This section draws heavily from Arnould, Rich and White (1993a).

4 There frequently is a US $10 copayment for certain services, e.g. for each visit to a participating HMO physician.

5 This section borrows heavily from Arnould et al (1993b) as well as the report by Arnould et al (1995). In addition, many of the ideas in this section are presented in Gift (1997).

6 There are also certain forms of indirect evidence that competition is having impacts on physicians similar to the impacts on hospitals. Hillman et al (1989) and DeBrock & Arnould (1992) provide evidence that the nature of the physician contract affects utilisation of hospital and physician services. Hillman et al (1989) found that salaried and capitated physicians utilised hospital and physician services at a significantly lower rate per enrollee than did those physicians paid on a fee for service or discounted fee for service basis. DeBrock & Arnould (1992) found that other elements in the contract such as the form of bonus and payback further influenced utilisation. They also found that these effects were significantly reduced in physician-owned HMOs where the physician presumably had more control over the method of reimbursement. Finally, Arnould & DeBrock (1995) found that the level of competition in the market had an influence over the ability of the HMO to negotiate contracts that passed more of the incentives to control utilisation on to physicians.

7 More evidence consistent with the hypothesis that competition is lowering costs and increasing efficiency in physician service markets is the impact competitive managed-care plans are having on incomes of physicians. Dranove et al (1992) found the incomes of specialists in California to be declining with the growth in managed-care programmes, which is consistent with expected effects of managed care, i.e. reductions in the price per unit, quantity of services provided or both. Similar results were found by Simon et al (1996).

8 Independent research by Hillman et al (1989) and DeBrock & Arnould (1992) reveals that a component of the savings being generated by competition in hospital markets results from conditions specified in the third-party-payer contract with physicians; i.e. physicians bear some of the responsibility for controlling hospital utilisation and reap some of the rewards for such success.

9 The methods used by Melnick et al (1992) to calculate hospital and ZIP code specific Hirschman–Herfindahl indices (HHI) are explained in Arnould et al (1995), Appendix A.

10 All of these percentages assume that no patients would react to higher prices by travelling outside the market area for hospital care; if any had done so, the increase in market concentration (and therefore prices) would have been smaller.

11 Ermann & Gabel (1986) use the definition for investor-owned hospital systems set by the American Hospital Association: 'three or more hospitals that are owned, managed, or leased by a single investor-owned organization'.

12 Refer to Mullner & Anderson (1987) and Brown & Klosterman (1986) for an analysis of the characteristics of merging firms.

13 The six conglomerates studied by Hoy & Gray (1986) were the Hospital Corporation of America, America Medical International, Humana, Inc., National Medial Enterprises, Charter Medical Corporation, and Republic Health Care Corporation.

14 Refer to Sloan et al (1987) for an analysis of capital market and multihospital systems.

15 Ermann & Gabel (1986) suggest the cost difference may be attributable to differences in system markups, more ancillary services being offered by systems, and/or newer and therefore more expensive facilities at system hospitals.

16 Watt et al (1986) address this question by examining the behaviour of systems after breaking them down by ownership status. Their results do not find significant cost differences between systems and independent hospitals when separated by IO and non-profit status. They offer the incentives from the Medicare reimbursement system as a possible explanation.

17 Reardon & Reardon (1995) p1065.
18 The concentration ratio measures what percentage of all yearly admissions occur in the four largest hospitals. Therefore, a concentration ratio of 25.5 means that the four largest hospitals in that urban area admitted 25.5 per cent of all patients in that year.
19 There is not a large body of literature addressing issues of quality and access with regard to hospital mergers. We will not delve into these issues here. The interested reader may refer to Shortell et al (1987) and Schlesinger et al (1987).
20 For example, if a merger announcement is made on 1 April and the event window is one week, stock values for rival firms will be recorded during the week prior to and following 1 April. These values are used to determine if there were abnormal stock returns for any of the rival firms which were caused by the event on 1 April.
21 For example: Firm A announces a merger in city 1; firm A competes with firm B in city 1 and city 2 and competes with firm C in cities 2, 3, and 4. Vita and Schumann would not have considered firm C to be a rival of firm A.
22 In this case, it is not enough to look merely at the prices charged by for-profit and non-profit hospitals. The literature on the differences between hospital prices for profit and non-profit institutions find that non-profit hospitals charge lower prices than for-profit hospitals. (For a review of empirical work in the area, see Lynk (1995a)). The presence of differential pricing between for-profit and non-profit hospitals is not enough to conclude that mergers will also have different effects. Even if non-profits have lower prices initially, they still may take advantage of increased market power and raise prices in the same manner as for-profit firms.
23 This summary taken from Bazzoli et al (1995). Refer to this work for further summary of the merger guidelines.
24 We do not discuss horizontal arrangements among buyers. The interested reader is referred to Havighurst (1995) and Eliasberg (1995).
25 See Arnould et al (1993b) for discussion of this point.
26 This does not include major metropolitan areas characterised as having small numbers of firms (hospitals).

[1] Although the Labour Government plans to replace the internal market (NHS Executive, 1997), it is nevertheless useful to examine the legal and accountability frameworks underpinning the purchaser–provider relationship, which it appears will be retained under future agreements for commissioning and delivering healthcare.

9

Different perspectives

9.1 THE LEGAL FRAMEWORK OF THE NHS INTERNAL MARKET[1]

Pauline Allen

9.1.1 Introduction

When analysing the market for healthcare in the United Kingdom, it is important to understand the extent to which most of this market is constituted by an internal market inside the National Health Service (NHS). This internal market was imposed on the centralised, publicly owned and run administrative system. Many aspects of this hierarchical system remain and the extent to which the present arrangements can be characterised as a market can be over-estimated. Consideration of the legal framework governing both the Trusts and the so-called 'contracts', which are at the core of the market, illustrate the point.

An internal market for certain types of community, secondary and tertiary healthcare was introduced by the National Health Service and Community Care Act 1990 (the 1990 Act) by means of a split between the purchasers of care and its providers. There are two categories of purchaser: district health authorities (DHAs) and certain 'fundholding' general practitioners (FHGPs). The remit of the DHAs is to purchase healthcare for their resident population with moneys which are allocated to them by central Government. FHGPs are given part of the budget for the DHA in which their practice is located. FHGPs use their budgets to purchase certain categories of non-urgent care for the patients registered with them. The providers of healthcare consist of 'self-governing Trusts', which have a special legal status within the

NHS. The theory is that Trusts must compete with each other to obtain funds from the purchasers. The arrangement made between purchasers and Trusts under which it is agreed what health services will be provided and at what price is referred to in the 1990 Act as a 'contract'.

9.1.2 Regulation of Trusts

In a private market, subject to certain laws (such as the Competition Act, 1980) concerning the abuse of monopoly power, firms are able to set their prices as they choose, in order to maximise the profit to be made by the sale of their goods and/or services. Each firm is also free to make decisions concerning the appropriate level of borrowing and other matters of financial planning and management. Although any firm will be constrained by the terms of any agreements reached with its lenders and shareholders, those terms will be the outcome of negotiation between those parties.

The legal regime governing the NHS internal market does not allow NHS Trusts such latitude, even though they are said to be 'operationally independent' (NHS Management Executive, 1990). These Trusts are *sui generis*, and certainly are not 'trusts' or 'charitable trusts' in the usual legal sense of the words. They are separately constituted entities, but do not have share capital and cannot, at present, be owned by the private sector. As the Trusts are still publicly owned, their financial affairs come within the constraints on all public sector organisations not to step outside the spending limits set by the Treasury. Section 10 of the 1990 Act explicitly states that: 'Every NHS trust shall ensure that its revenue is not less than sufficient, taking one financial year with another, to meet outgoings properly chargeable to revenue account [and it] shall be the duty of every NHS trust to achieve such financial objectives as may from time to time be set by the Secretary of State with consent of the Treasury and as are applicable to it ...' These objectives include an obligation on Trusts to make a return of 6 per cent per annum on their net assets. The NHS Executive will set a cash limit for each Trust on net external borrowings for each financial year (the External Financing Limit) and, in any event, prior approval is required for substantial borrowing.

Furthermore, detailed administrative guidance has been issued by the centre directing that prices must be based on average costs (marginal costs can only be used for unplanned spare capacity in excess of assumed volumes of service and must only be applied during that actual financial year in which the spare capacity arose). There can be no cross-subsidisation from one contract, procedure or specialty to another using prices. Differential tariffs cannot be offered by a provider to different purchasers, despite the fact that they may be buying very different quantities of services. Dawson (1994) has argued that the model of the NHS internal market used by the National Steering Group on Costing (which formulated the guidelines) is inappropriate for the type of market to be found in the NHS.

The effect of these constraints on Trusts is to ensure that the internal market will not operate in the same way a 'conventional' market would. It is a managed market. The extent to which the internal market is managed was made more explicit by the issuing of administrative guidelines, 'The Operation of the NHS Internal Market: Local Freedoms, National Responsibilities' (NHS Executive, 1994). These are in addition to the legal framework set out in the 1990 Act and are an attempt to replace the previous *ad hoc* approach to regulation with a more rule-based approach. Their issue illustrates the extent of administrative involvement in the market, which they attempt to codify. (The guidelines deal with the circumstances in which the NHS Executive intends to intervene in local affairs in respect of the following five situations: provider mergers and joint ventures; purchaser joint ventures; purchaser mergers and boundary adjustments; providers in financial difficulties; and collusion between providers and between purchasers and providers. The guidelines are designed to promote the competitive structure of the market and to mitigate the effects of lack of competition.) Despite this attempt to regularise administrative involvement in the internal market it is clear that political considerations are often of overriding importance. Indeed the guidelines acknowledge that the final decision in respect of mergers, for example, rests with ministers, and that non-economic considerations, such as 'retaining units which are popular with the public' (p12) are an important consideration.

9.1.3 'Contracts'

The tight legislative framework in respect of NHS internal market 'contracts' is particularly pertinent when demonstrating how this market differs from a private market.

The obligation to make 'contracts' in the NHS internal market has been imposed on all DHAs by the provisions of the 1990 Act. It is a prerequisite of a legally binding contract that each party enter into the agreement of its own free will. Contracts must be voluntary agreements made by free agents, in order to be recognised by the law. The right not to enter into a contract is an essential aspect of the rule of law. This is because, if they did not have the right to refuse to enter into a contract, the weak would be exposed to the arbitrary and compulsory imposition of obligations by the strong, who would receive the backing of the State (in the shape of the courts) to enforce them. (The point of making a legally binding contract is that, ultimately, the courts will enforce one's rights enshrined in that contract.) Although it is only the *process* of contracting which has been imposed on the NHS institutions by the Government, not the actual parties with whom agreements must be made, there may be little choice of contractual partner in many circumstances. It is for this reason that the powers to protect the 'weak' (discussed below) were conferred on the Secretary of State. Although GPs would seem to have more freedom than DHAs to decide whether to enter into 'contracts', because they can decide whether to apply for fundholding status or not, once a GP has decided to become a fundholder, they are obliged to purchase the range of services covered by the type of fundholding scheme they have joined.

There is another way in which the formation of NHS 'contracts' differs significantly from that of legally binding commercial contracts. It is axiomatic in classical legal doctrine that the parties to a contract are free to make any bargain they choose. (In fact, over the years various legal fetters on such freedom have developed, such as the Unfair Contract Terms Act 1977). Subject to certain exceptions, mainly designed to protect consumers, parties to contracts are left to come to an agreement which is the result of negotiation.

By contrast, the 1990 Act provides that if the two prospective parties to an NHS 'contract' cannot agree the terms of the 'contract' during their negotiations, because of any reason arising out of their relative bargaining positions, either such party can refer the matter to the Secretary of State for Health 'who may specify terms to be included in the proposed arrangement and may direct that it be proceeded with' (Section 4(6)). The NHS Management Executive, issued guidance on resolving disputes (NHS Management Executive, 1991) which directed potential parties to take their disputes to their regional health authority for informal conciliation before the formal procedure in the 1990 Act is invoked. The guidance also explained that an adjudicator appointed by the Secretary of State would regard an unequal bargaining position as existing if 'either a purchaser threatened to cease securing services, or a provider threatened to cease supplying them, if its terms were not agreed, in circumstances where no alternative practical provider or purchaser was available.' This possibility of pre-'contractual' intervention as to the actual terms of the agreement amounts to the imposition of a 'contract' on the parties and, as such, is unprecedented in the arena of legally enforceable contracts. In the commercial world, if firms cannot reach agreement, each is free to 'walk away' from the other and to refuse to contract at all. Indeed, there may well be circumstances when the terms available indicate that it would not be cost-effective for a particular firm to do business with the other party to the proposed contract. This situation cannot be allowed to occur in the NHS internal market because of the political obligation to ensure the delivery of services to the entire population.

The possibility of the *imposition* of a 'contract', ultimately by the Secretary of State, may well have the effect of inducing parties in strong bargaining positions to refrain from 'abusing' those positions and imposing disadvantageous terms on the other party. If this is the case, it can be argued that this statutory provision will make the internal market work better than it would otherwise do, because any inefficiencies due to any lack of competition between providers are being vitiated by this fetter on the abuse of monopoly power provided in the 1990 Act. There is no publicly available evidence that any pre-'contractual' disputes have been referred to the Secretary of State. It is clear, however, that regional offices of the NHS Executive (which superseded regional health authorities in 1995) have been acting as informal 'conciliators' in these circumstances. There does not appear to be any available systematic evidence about the actual effect of these frequent interventions (confusingly and erroneously referred to by staff in the NHS as 'arbitration'). Anecdotally, it appears that these 'conciliations' are mostly in respect of disputes about the allocation of limited resources to different parts of the NHS system.

Hughes et al have suggested (1994) that these frequent pre-'contractual' interventions by (what were then) regional health authorities are not about the setting of the terms of a 'contract', but fundamentally about strategic planning and resource allocation. Thus, the hierarchical aspects of the administrative system are clearly in evidence. 'The issue is not about authoritative interpretation but the pragmatic settlement of complex problems' (p17). They argue that it is appropriate for this type of problem to be dealt with in the informal setting of regional conciliation, where management directions can be issued to the parties and the multiple aspects of the problem can be considered, rather than as a formal adversarial process in which only the arguments of the two parties present are considered as competing claims of rights or accusations of fault, on which the adjudicator must reach a principled judgement. This view of pre-'contractual' conciliation is linked to the views of Hughes & Dingwall (1990) that instead of the 1990 Act having introduced a market of any kind, 'the use of internal contracts will simply introduce an alternative rule-based system of governance that is both more specific and more difficult to enforce' (p306).

It is an essential attribute of an ordinary commercial contract that it is enforceable by the State at the behest of any of the contracting parties. In contrast, the 1990 Act provides that an NHS 'contract' 'shall not be regarded for any purpose as giving rise to contractual rights or liabilities, but if any dispute arises with respect to such an arrangement, either party may refer the matter to the Secretary of State for determination' (Section 4(3)). This is intended to ensure that the resolution of any dispute between the parties is kept out of the courts. Such matters must be kept within the control of the politically run administrative system. The 1990 Act allows the determination of a reference to the Secretary of State to include 'such directions as the Secretary of State... considers appropriate to resolve the matter in dispute' (Section 4(7)). These powers are explicitly deemed to include the possibility of varying the terms of the 'contract' or terminating it (Section 4(8)). The latitude given to the Secretary of State by the foregoing is considerably wider than the principles which govern the resolution of real contractual disputes by the courts. A court must interpret the agreement that was made by the parties at the time the contract was entered into. It cannot impose some other terms on them, however unfair those terms might appear later. (In fact, this classical legal rule has been tempered by the invention of a range of mechanisms, such as promissory estoppel, which allow a more equitable solution to be reached in some circumstances. These developments in the law can be seen as part of the decline of the strictly classical, liberal doctrine of contract (see Attiyah, 1979). In fact, it is questionable whether the parties to many long-term contracts resort to the letter of the contract when many types of disputes arise (Allen, 1995)).

Despite the wide powers given to the Secretary of State by the 1990 Act, the NHS Management Executive issued guidelines stating that the principles to be applied in resolving disputes between parties to NHS 'contracts' should recognise the concept of freedom of contract. 'The presumption in determining a dispute is likely to be that the outcome will give effect to the agreement which was originally reached, rather than a new agreement which the parties should have reached' (NHS Management Executive, 1991).

Disputes which are referred to the Secretary of State will be subject to The National Health Service Contracts (Dispute Resolution) Regulations (SI 1996/623), in which it is stipulated that the adjudicator appointed by the Secretary of State must give reasons for his decision. Such decisions will be subject to judicial review by the court, and if this were to occur, it would encourage a clear set of principles to emerge as to how such decisions are to be made. There is no publicly available evidence that any such judicial review proceedings have taken place.

It is thought (in the absence of any centralised reporting) that very few disputes concerning the terms of concluded NHS 'contracts' have been referred to the Secretary of State. The report from an arbitrator appointed in respect of a dispute in Wales suggests that, once again, the dispute actually concerned the initial failure to make the allocation of moneys explicit, rather than any allegations of failure to perform the terms of the 'contract' (personal communication from the arbitrator, 1996). However, disputes have been referred to regional health authorities, for informal arbitration. It has been reported by Appleby (1994) that in 1992/3 20 per cent of providers and 30 per cent of DHAs surveyed used arbitration, though the type of arbitration was not specified and may include both pre- and post-'contractual' disputes. As informal arbitration is probably not subject to judicial review, and it is being encouraged in the place of referral to the Secretary of State, it is likely that no consistent principles concerning the exercise of the power to resolve disputes will emerge. Anecdotal evidence suggests that these disputes also concern the allocation of resources. In one case, pre-'contractual' conciliation was required to agree the global sum payable by a DHA to a local Trust, and later in the financial year, post-'contractual' conciliation was required as the original settlement had not been articulated explicitly enough for both parties to agree what had been decided. In fact, no written record of the original, pre-contractual, conciliation had

been produced (personal communication from contracting manager, 1996).

There is some debate as to whether the provisions of section 4(3) of the 1990 Act will be effective in preventing the court from adjudicating in the event of a dispute involving an NHS 'contract'. Jacob (1991) suggests various legal mechanisms which might allow the court to assume jurisdiction in such a case. These include the possibility of an action for a *quantum meruit* (which is a right, outside the law of contract, to be paid for work undertaken). Jacob suggests there may also be methods allowing individual citizens to question the terms of the 'contract' or how it has been performed. None of these appears to have been tested in the courts.

Thus the regime affecting the resolution of disputes arising out of NHS 'contracts' differs from that which pertains to ordinary contracts. It is not clear what principles will be applied when a dispute requires resolution. This makes the task of drafting the 'contracts' difficult because it is not known whether they will be interpreted as ordinary contracts (whether by the Secretary of State, regional offices of the NHS Executive or the courts) or whether a wider view will be taken of the arbitrator's powers to alter the original terms. As ordinary contracts are subject to the ultimate jurisdiction of the courts, consistent principles of interpretation have developed which enable those drafting the documents to do so with some certainty as to the implications of the provisions made. This cannot be said to apply inside the NHS internal market.

9.1.4 Effect on concentration and choice

The foregoing examples of the legal regime in respect of NHS trusts and 'contracts' demonstrates the extent to which the NHS internal market retains the character of a centralised, politically-influenced administrative hierarchy. In such a system, issues related to market concentration, such as mergers of providers and the creation (or *de facto* existence) of supplier monopolies at local level, will always be subject to overriding political considerations. Indeed, the administrative guidelines (NHSE, 1991) make this explicit. The assumption in the guidelines is that the Competition Act 1980, which requires the referral of potentially anti-competitive problems of market concentration to the independent Monopolies and Mergers Commission, does not apply to the NHS internal market. Dawson (1995) argues that there is an inherent conflict of interest between the Department of Health's role in rationalising capacity in the NHS and the enforcement of competition policy, which requires the maintenance of excess capacity and new entry.

The structure of NHS 'contracts', to which no actual patient is a party, demonstrates the lack of individual choice introduced by the internal market. 'Contracts' are made by FHGPs or DHAs, acting as agents for patients. The economic theory of such agency relationships states that there will be problems in aligning the acts (and incentives) of agents with the wishes of their (diverse) principals (Guesnerie, 1989). NHS bodies are not agents of individuals in the legal meaning of the term 'agent', as there is no legally binding contract of agency between them. Accountability for decisions by these 'agents' is (in the case of FHGPs) via 'exit' from their service, and (in the case of DHAs) via the political process and the usual remedies of public law. The latter are mainly concerned with procedural issues concerning *how* a decision is made, rather than the content of the decision.

9.1.5 Conclusion

The legal structure of the NHS internal market is far removed from that of private markets. Nevertheless, it should be noted that not all healthcare in the United Kingdom is purchased through this mechanism. There is a significant private sector for the provision of some surgical specialties in some areas (for example, elective surgery for prostate problems in the London area) to which the constraints set out above do not apply. Furthermore, the system of law described above is not immutable: it can be changed as quickly as the original legislation introducing the internal market was made.

9.2 ACCOUNTABILITY AND HEALTHCARE MARKETS[1]

Justin Keen

9.2.1 Introduction

The introduction of policies designed to create managed markets and competition raises questions about accountability. Traditionally, the main accountability mechanisms for the NHS were 'vertical', from the ward and the surgery to professional bodies, to the Department of Health and to Parliament. Changes in the structure and financing of the NHS over the last two decades have, though, complicated the picture. The creation of an internal market, with regulation of some aspects of its operation, means that the hierarchical model of vertical accountability has been overlaid by the purchaser-provider relationship. In addition, successive Government policies have promoted more localised accountability relationships, and the notion of accountability of professionals to the patients they care for has come to greater prominence. Different forms of accountability therefore co-exist within the NHS, and merit examination.

This section outlines the nature of the arrangements for ensuring accountability of the NHS to Parliament for its use of resources, highlights the main elements of the changes in structures and financing which influence these accountability arrangements, and discusses some of the implications of these changes.

9.2.2 Concepts of vertical accountability

Concepts of accountability within public services have evolved over time. When the NHS was founded the belief was that there should be a clear line of accountability from service providers to ministers. Aneurin Bevan's dictum (see Foot, 1973), that 'every time a maid kicks over a bucket of slops in a ward an agonised wail will go through Whitehall', captures this concept. Day and Klein (1987) argued that there were really many different accountability relationships from the start, and by the 1980s it was clear that Bevan's view had become outdated, and vertical accountability had been overlaid by the complex accountability relationships associated with a modern health service. Older notions of public accountability which focused mainly on political and financial affairs were broadened in the process, so that, for example, patients (as 'customers') are now in principle able to hold service providers to account. However, cases that achieve national importance, such as that of 'Child B' or tragedies in Accident and Emergency Departments, remind us that vertical relationships still exist: Members of Parliament still play a role in these events.

One of the key vertical mechanisms is concerned with financial accountability, and has evolved over a period of more than a century. At its apex is the Committee of Public Accounts of the House of Commons, which was formed in the middle of the nineteenth century. The Comptroller and Auditor General reports to the Committee: formerly supported by the Exchequer and Audit Department, since 1983 he has been supported by the National Audit Office (NAO). The NAO audits the accounts of government departments (including the Department of Health), agencies and other public bodies. It also publishes some 50 Value For Money studies each year, the majority of which are considered by the Committee. A proportion of these Value For Money reports are about the work of the NHS, recent examples being a progress report on the Health of the Nation (NAO, 1996a), NHS Supplies (NAO, 1996b) and Health and Safety (NAO, 1996c). Senior officials give evidence to the Committee of Public Accounts about reports, making them directly accountable to Parliament for the ways in which they have discharged their financial responsibilities.

The vertical accountability relationship is still developing, with the NAO and other bodies having to respond to major changes in the organisation of public services, and policy makers having to work out the consequences of the new structures for governance and for accountability relationships. Who should hold whom to account, for what actions, and according to what criteria? The issue in the first years of the new NHS market structure was to reconcile the devolved responsibility of local managers and local markets with the requirement for the service as a whole – and in particular the NHS Chief Executive – to remain accountable to Parliament for the proper use of NHS resources. In 1994, the NHS Executive issued a new Code of Conduct and Accountability to the Service with the aim of clarifying the responsibilities of Chief Executives and their Boards. In terms of financial accountability to Parliament, the NHS Executive has placed a specific responsibility on Chief Executives at local level to be accountable for their stewardship of public funds. They are accountable in the first instance to the Executive and ultimately, via the NHS Chief Executive, to Parliament. In this way it is intended that vertical accountability, at least on detailed issues of financial stewardship, should complement rather than inhibit local decision making and accountabilities.

9.2.3 Changes in structure and process

The policy changes in the NHS can usefully be viewed as a particular instance of major changes being initiated across the UK public sector and in the public sectors in many developed countries (Pollitt, 1993). These changes have attracted different labels, including the New Public Management in the UK (Dunleavy & Hood, 1994) and Re-inventing Government in the USA (Osborne & Gaebler, 1992). At base they embody a belief in the virtues of private-sector practices, seeking either to replicate aspects of the behaviour of private firms, or to enable private firms themselves to deliver services. In implementation, however, it has become clear that private-sector concepts have to be adapted to the particular circumstances of public-service delivery. Lowndes (1996) notes that it is difficult to identify clear conceptual frameworks that underpin the changes in any one area of Government, and no public service has been designed according to a single identifiable model or body of theory. The result is that key mechanisms such as those operating in quasi-markets are novel and as yet not well understood. Further, the extent to which these structural changes have led to real process change on the ground is unclear. Reviewing the evidence, Ferlie et al (1996) suggest that real change has occurred but has been patchy, both in the type of change that has occurred and in the variation between different parts of the UK. The overall picture is therefore one of new modes of service delivery which are not well explained by existing theories, whose implementation is patchy, and which are developing over time.

One result of these changes is that arrangements for regulation, monitoring and inspection of the work of the NHS are also developing. In the NHS, factors such as a powerful medical profession and tight Treasury and Department of Health spending controls mean that the character of these models will differ from those developed for, say, the privatised utilities. At the risk of simplifying the debate here, it is useful to distinguish two broad forms of regulation, namely economic and social (Ogus, 1994), relating to individuals as economic actors and as social actors respectively. For economic regulation, the NHS Executive is responsible for regulation of the internal market, including purchaser and provider mergers, collusion and providers who get into financial difficulties. Dawson (1995) noted the duality of the Regulator's role in managing rationalization of capacity (e.g. in service mergers) and enforcing competition policy, and argues that there are tensions inherent in the arrangement.

The need to resolve arrangements for regulation and accountability is highlighted in the cases of closure and merger of services. Some proposals have been re-thought or abandoned in the face of sustained local campaigns, which emphasises the point that local service users and affected staff are stakeholders. On the one hand, then, there are arguments for decisions to be made locally, following appropriate consultation. On the other hand there would certainly appear to be a role for a regulator, who may wish to investigate whether a merger or closure might be against the public interest, just as the Monopolies and Mergers Commission might investigate mergers or takeovers involving private firms. The arrangements for reconciling the different preferences of the various local stakeholders with one another and with those of the Regulator remain to be settled.

Arrangements for social regulation – which broadly focus on consumer-protection issues – have developed along different lines to economic regulation, with policies tending to favour low-level central intervention. An important complication here is the relatively weak relationship between managers and doctors – and to a lesser extent other service providers – which limits the extent to which the former can hold the latter to account for the quality of their work. (This seems still to be true in spite of a number of developments, including the creation of clinical directorates and the introduction of clinical audit, which hints at the possibility that they may be more symbolic than substantial in many places.) Arguably, one driver of many recent policies is the desire of ministers and civil servants to make doctors more manageable, by emphasising accountability to colleagues and to patients. The result is that different policies for social regulation co-exist alongside one another. In short, it is possible to say that:

- useful theory and solid empirical evidence about key mechanisms such as the operation of quasi-markets and regulation are still lacking;
- there are tensions and inconsistencies in the purchaser–provider relationship – which may to some extent be inevitable – and there may therefore be risks to efficiency and effectiveness.

These points have implications for vertical accountability arrangements.

9.2.4 Implications for audit scrutiny

In 'The Operation of the NHS Internal Market: Local Freedoms, National Responsibilities' (1994), the NHS Executive cited the creation of the purchaser–provider relationship as the key spur to improved efficiency. Taken together with the Code of Conduct and Accountability, the new arrangements emphasise a 'mixed model' with a number of different relationships and types of accountability co-existing. Even if one considers only financial accountability, mainly conducted through financial and Value For Money audits, there are a number of relationships involved: while the NAO is responsible for reporting to Parliament, the Audit Commission and District Audit Service have responsibilities for the audit of NHS Trusts and other local bodies. Increasingly, the availability of evidence about the clinical effectiveness and cost-effectiveness of treatments raises questions about who is responsible for ensuring that best practices are observed. If one accepts that the 'mixed model' is here to stay, there are issues concerning the ways in which accountability to Parliament might work. Three issues are highlighted here, namely the scrutiny of accountability to other stakeholders, of the market mechanism itself, and the work of the NHS Executive.

Scrutiny of accountability to other stakeholders

One of the stated aims of the NHS internal market is to make services more responsive – and more accountable – to patients and to local communities. Evidence about these issues is patchy, but Mays and Dixon (1996) suggest that there is cause for concern in the emerging models of purchasing, where there are different forms of relationship between GPs and health authorities. They point to the potential conflicts of interest in the dual role of GPs as purchasers and providers of services, and note that where purchasing decisions have been devolved to GPs, governance and accountability structures are currently under-developed. This is one example of a situation where local accountability relationships may be weak, and where there may be a role for Parliament in examining the efficacy of local accountability relationships or the strength of accountability to Parliament itself. (Who else, one might ask, can realistically hold GPs to account?)

Scrutiny of the market mechanism

There are two key questions about market mechanisms that an auditor body might ask.

The first question concerns the proper conduct of public business: are NHS staff behaving in ways expected of employees in public services (see Committee of Public Accounts 1994)? A 'hands-off' style of management may increase the risk of opportunistic behaviour, and it may be necessary to investigate specific instances. A well-known example in the NHS is the failure of the Wessex Regional Information Systems Plan, which was investigated first by the District Auditor, then reported on to Parliament; a critical report was published by the Committee (Committee of Public Accounts, 1993).

The second question is about the operation of the market, including the extent to which service mergers increase efficiency, and whether purchasers are in practice able to promote competition. Treasury and Department of Health spending controls notwithstanding, there may be important financial risks associated with existing arrangements. As earlier chapters have emphasised, there are methods available for analysing the extent of competition in a given locality, but also important technical problems that have to be solved in undertaking studies and interpreting data. Making even high-level judgements about the performance of the NHS will require substantial amounts of data about costs, volume and outcomes. At least at present appropriate data are not available to do this, as national data sets focus more on the overall performance of individual bodies than on the efficiency and effectiveness of internal market mechanisms. As a result, data that would allow assessment of whether service mergers have led to efficiency gains are not generally available. If Parliament – or anyone else – wishes to know about specific aspects of purchaser– provider relationships it is still necessary to go into the NHS to obtain and interpret data, it, and bodies such as the NAO have the legal powers to do so.

In time, it is likely that better performance management data will become available. This might include hospital mortality rates, certain contracts based on Healthcare Related Groups (HRG) data, and more reliable resource use data. The result may be more 'transparent' individual Trusts and other NHS bodies, which become easier to audit. Reports on NHS activity might look like financial accounts in some respects. Reports to Parliament and other external stakeholders might therefore change in form, perhaps relying more on performance indicators than they do now. This said, it is also likely that contracting and regulation will become more technical in nature, not least because the same performance indicators will make it possible to scrutinise behaviour in more detail than before, and contractors or regulators can apply incentive-based and other instruments to solve problems they identify. The result may therefore be that the focus of audit develops over time, to include scrutiny of these new instruments and their effects.

Scrutiny of the work of the NHS Executive

Dawson's (1995) observation that there may be tensions between the management and regulatory roles of the NHS Executive suggests that there are questions about the work of the Executive itself. There is therefore a need to monitor the developing arrangements for managing and regulating the NHS, and if necessary scrutinise the effectiveness of the NHS Executive in carrying out its functions. It has proved possible to scrutinise utilities regulators' use of licence conditions, rules about the design of contracts and other strategies to achieve stated objectives (see for example NAO, 1996d), so the NHS Executive should be amenable to analysis.

9.2.5 Conclusions

This section has argued that the new NHS structures have implications for vertical accountability. There are new structures to report on, and complex new mechanisms to scrutinise.

The arguments suggest that vertical accountability remains important and can be summarised as follows:

* The NHS remains a predominantly publicly-funded and delivered service, and so accountability to Parliament is still appropriate;

* Parliament still becomes involved in NHS issues such as rationing and hospital closures – so there are occasions when the bucket's echo still reaches Westminster;
* the new structures are innovative, and create new types of financial and other risk, and Parliament is well placed to consider NHS-wide issues such as the efficiency of purchaser–provider relationships;
* issues surrounding the appropriateness and strength of more local accountability mechanisms, and the extent to which the NHS Executive can resolve tensions within its role, are still unclear.

To set against these arguments, the sheer complexity of the NHS means that vertical accountability alone is not enough – indeed, it never has been. The problem at present is that more localised accountability relationships are not well defined, and there are gaps and inconsistencies. The task for the future, then, is to arrive at arrangements that reflect the interests of the many local and national stakeholders involved. As understanding develops, so the merits of each form of accountability will become clearer.

9.3 CHANGING SERVICE CONFIGURATION: A PURCHASER'S PERSPECTIVE

Jane Eminson

A purchaser's first task when alterations to the concentration or choice of healthcare services are suggested is to analyse quickly but accurately the reasons why the question has been asked and who is driving the change. Challenges to existing service configurations can come from a whole variety of sources. Clinical quality or medical staffing concerns are usually behind regional and national pressure for change, sometimes with the added flavour of 'you won't be able to afford to carry on as you are now'. The evidence base for the type of question which deals with clinical quality may not stand up to the type of rigorous evaluation which the *Effective Health Care* Bulletins undertake. It commonly has national or Royal

College backing, however, and therefore cannot be ignored by local purchasers.

More local questions arise from financial comparisons such as 'why do we spend so much on ...?' or 'why are the prices so high for ...,' followed immediately by uncertainty over the information used and the validity of the comparison. Reconfiguration of neighbouring services can have consequences (foreseen or unforeseen) for local health care and can, therefore, raise concerns. Local political pressure is another source of challenge to existing service patterns where inadequacies are perceived. Combinations of the Community Health Council, specialist interest groups, local consultants and MPs can sometimes come together and bring about a seemingly irresistible momentum for change, usually founded on access or quality concerns or both. (Such alliances can on other occasions form an equally powerful resistance to change.) Occasionally purchaser monitoring of access or quality leads to a service configuration question but this is rare in the absence of other drivers.

Analysing the pressure for change is important because a good understanding will ensure that an appropriate analysis is carried out and may determine the approach to evaluating options. At this stage it is also crucial to decide whether or not the question is 'real' and what priority it should have. For example, some medical staffing threats to service configurations are very real while others simply result in imaginative solutions by providers which remove the need for further consideration for the foreseeable future. A priority judgement is crucial because a lot of work and uncertainty for those delivering and receiving services can be saved by deciding early on that service change is a low priority or unlikely to yield significant benefits. Doing the work and deciding later on a 'no change' option is often damaging to purchaser credibility. An early quick and dirty desk-top exercise is essential if these pitfalls are to be avoided.

For those who decide to continue with a review of service configurations, the conclusions of the *Effective Health Care* Bulletin on volume, cost and quality are supported by experience. In particular, the inadequacies of routine hospital data when adjusting for casemix are repeatedly a major stumbling block in analyses of the need for change or of service options. Differences between providers in counting and coding are often so great that they completely alter the results of the analysis. This problem gets worse when costed comparisons are attempted. The costing of services and especially of HRGs still involves so much apportionment that, at best, comparisons may not stand up to scrutiny and, at worst, they may be meaningless.

There are several key factors which are missing, however, from a theoretical analysis of service configuration issues – for example, whether the change is within a single Trust or involves more than one organisation, the influence of consultants and the impact of alterations in clinical practice. Even the cost of change, which is part of the standard option appraisal process, can be missed in practice: for example, the capital charges bill and the exit costs have a habit of creeping up, apparently reasonably, after a change has been agreed.

Achieving service change within a single Trust is usually much easier than if other Trusts are involved. This is especially true if the income to the Trust is guaranteed by an agreement that savings generated will be used for the development of another service. Local opinion formers, especially users of the service and their carers, should be actively involved in the analysis and the consideration of options and are ignored at your peril. There is usually adequate information to demonstrate the financial or quality benefits of the change, comparisons are rarely required, and a well-managed process should result in an improved service within a reasonable timescale. Examples here are rationalisation of the number of sites over which a service is delivered or changing the access criteria. Even changes within a Trust can, however, sometimes give nasty surprises. Planners of the move of a local accident and emergency department by about one mile noticed only late in the day that, according to existing ambulance routing criteria, the catchment area for the new site was significantly larger than the old.

Changes involving more than one Trust are more difficult and are greatly affected by the attitude of managers and clinicians in the Trusts concerned. In practice, the way to achieve these changes quickly is to guarantee the income to each Trust for use on other services or for other cost pressures. This is difficult if the major driver of change is the need to make financial savings, but can produce a solution with a recurring financial balance even if there are non-recurring problems.

Consultants gain a further dimension of influence when they work across more than one Trust. It is not uncommon, especially in smaller specialties, for different options to be evaluated where the same consultants are involved in more than one proposal. Shared appointments, of course, can be an excellent way to reach efficient volume/cost thresholds. It is also important to remember that clinical perspectives on the type of service needed can vary tremendously, and the path through the different views is difficult for Health Authorities as the necessary expert advice is not usually available in-house. There seem to be two 'facts of life' about professional advice. First, the local consultant who is receptive to an external adviser is usually the one whose perspective agrees with the literature and written 'expert' sources. Conversely, the consultant who is resistant to external advice may well be in the specialty with a large diversity of views. Second, the more advice you take the higher will be the final quality specification and the more the service will cost.

The cost to the purchaser of changing a service configuration is rarely mentioned. The initial analysis may stretch the capacity of Health Authorities and Trusts and therefore consultancy costs may be incurred. If tendering is decided upon it is necessary to prepare the specification, invite submissions and set up an evaluation process. All of these will involve additional costs, which can be substantial. A commonly held view is that tendering for clinical services results in choosing the Trust that you initially wanted to provide the service but at a cost greater than you originally wanted to pay. Changing a service always seems to result in a quality specification higher than that of the existing service being adopted, usually with associated costs. Additionally, moving a service may result in staff redundancies and other exit costs which may wipe out savings for several years. The impact of the new service on access rates is also usually under-estimated, especially if the new service is more locally accessible, because the extent of unmet demand hidden by the previous less satisfactory service is difficult to estimate. The final factor which adds to the cost of change is that the new improved service always seems to have the effect of raising activity levels in some area that was not considered in the initial analysis. For example, with hindsight it is very easy to say, 'Why didn't we consider the impact on physiotherapy or diagnostic services of moving the rheumatology service to the local provider?' Some of these additional costs are non-recurring or have a limited life, but the overall effect can all too easily be to reduce substantially the expected savings. These additional costs may be met by increased provider efficiency, purchaser investment or a combination of both. Whatever approach to funding is adopted will, of course, incur an opportunity cost.

Changes in clinical practice can be dramatic and are rarely adequately reflected in contractual arrangements until some time after the event. Such changes can have several effects on service-configuration discussions. First, they add to the initial analytical problems: 'We must remember to adjust the data for the open-access gynaecology clinic/varicose veins/low back pain service ...', and, second, they undermine the robustness of the conclusions especially when a change in clinical practice is already known about: 'What effect will the increasingly medical treatment of prostate disease have on referral and operation rates for urology ...?' A final cautionary note in relation to clinical practice is the unpredictability of GP referral patterns. Sometimes these change very quickly but on other occasions GPs stay with the same provider despite an easily available and apparently better quality service elsewhere. The reasons why this is so are unclear but it seems that any change in service configuration must be supported by the provision of good quality information to GPs (and general dental practitioners) if any expected change in referral patterns is to materialise.

Discussions about changing services also

have an impact on the behaviour of Trusts. There is a definite Hawthorne Effect in relation to analyses of service configurations. In the face of a perceived threat to a service, a Trust can move very quickly either to improve its efficiency or to attract more patients to the service so that it is no longer in danger. Some of the changes may be desirable but others may not and all of these can seriously cloud the analysis and evaluation of options: 'What under-used dermatology beds are you talking about? . . . Have you seen our new sleep apnoea centre?'

Such cautionary tales are to be learnt from and do not detract from the value of looking at questions of concentration and choice in health care. They lead to conclusions about the approach to this work which I hope may have some relevance to other people involved in such exercises. My apologies if the following conclusions seem trite or obvious.

First, analysis and evaluation of service configurations is not yet an exact science. Scientifically rigorous analysis must be supplemented by a wide range of evidence, opinion and judgement. Only when this range of results yields a consistent answer is a change likely to be achieved and result in an improved service. Second, do not start with a purchaser review of the service. If the Trusts concerned work with local GPs, service users, carers and Community Health Council representatives (with purchaser involvement), the outcome is again likely to be an improvement in care. Appropriate and sensitive leadership of such work, especially if more than one Trust is involved, is naturally very important and needs careful consideration by all concerned. Third, ensure that the work is set within a clear and cautious financial framework from the beginning. This will avoid unnecessarily raising expectations and should result in an improved service which is also affordable.

9.4 REFLECTIONS OF AN NHS TRUST CHIEF EXECUTIVE

Peter Kennedy

I write from the perspective of a Chief Executive of a large Whole District Trust, with just over £100 million turnover per annum. We have 103 Consultants and 3,500 staff (WTEs). The acute hospital was built for 800 beds and 25,000 admissions a year. It now uses about 650 beds for 40,000 in-patient and 18,000 day cases. A large rural area surrounds us with three smaller Whole District Trusts within 20 miles and two large teaching hospitals 30 miles away. One Health Authority accounts for 65 per cent of our income. Most general practitioners in the area are fundholders.

9.4.1 Clinging to the status quo

The NHS internal market commenced in the early 1990s with paranoia in smaller Trusts that large Trusts would be predatory. So nothing much happened at first. The only 'deal' I was offered was to help another Trust block the loss of its ENT services to a Teaching Hospital. My Trust would gain a little income in the process. Since the proposal was to cling on to income without addressing the quality problems of a single consultant specialty, it did not seem to be worth the bother. It would not last. There was no pressure for change from the increasing number of GP fundholders. Most told the Health Authority that they would prefer the status quo, with small specialties in every DGH. Some said they would oppose change even if presented with evidence of inferior outcomes and higher mortalities. No one bothered to raise such questions with patients or the public.

9.4.2 Necessity concentrates minds

Subsequently the pressures built up on smaller DGHs. Colleges and postgraduate deans have threatened or actually withdrawn accreditation for junior doctor training. Health Authorities pushed for increasing sub-specialisation. Small consultant firms could not sub-specialise and at the same time provide the range of supervised experience for juniors. Now our main Health Authority is quite explicit in wanting its services provided by specialties with no less than three consultants and preferably four. NCEPOD reports followed up by National Audits have given further impetus to the requirement for larger consultant teams because of demonstrably higher perioperative mortality and morbidity for emergency procedures carried out by unsupervised juniors.

Necessity began to foster a spirit of collaboration. Shared services were better than no income and service at all. Thus two small Trusts sought partnership with my Trust to develop several small surgical and medical specialties (Oral Surgery, ENT, Urology, Neurology, Dermatology and Rheumatology). We employ the consultants in teams of three or more with junior and middle-grade cover. They accept that the more complex in-patient treatments are provided in York. We guarantee that those parts of the service which could be provided locally will be. Our consultants have sessions in these other Trusts seeing out-patients, doing day treatments and consulting on their wards. Such an approach recognises the need for critical mass in delivering high-tech treatments (concentration), along with the convenience of local services wherever possible (choice).

And so over the last three years centralisation of the high-tech aspects of the smaller specialties has started to roll forward in collaborative partnerships between Trusts. My own Trust has been a gainer in terms of volume and range of services (43 per cent increase in consultant establishment). I would like to think that we have expanded because we are excellent, but I think there are other important factors in our favour, like geographical location and accessibility. We were to begin with the biggest DGH in the County. York is a nice place to live so recruitment is easier. Whilst other Trusts were becoming desperate about consultant vacancies in Anaesthetics, Psychiatry and various surgical specialties, we had plenty of good applicants.

9.4.3 Patient power

More recently we have started to gain services as the local 'spoke' of a tertiary-service 'hub' in the Teaching Centres. Patient choice and convenience does seem to have been an important influence here. Patients requiring chronic renal dialysis have been vociferous in wanting this to be provided in York rather than in Leeds. The Health Authority has been impressed that we can offer a better price. Delay is being caused

by the difficulty of prising the money out of the losing tertiary centre, understandably very concerned about being left with fixed and semi fixed costs. Health Authorities need to reserve bridging funds to give losing providers more time to reduce their costs.

There are welcome signs that professionals are increasingly sensitive to patient pressure for change in the provision of cancer services. The Calman plan for Cancer Units and Cancer Centres seems to be moving faster than most national policies in the past. Powerful TV programmes and influential women's magazines have alerted the public to the fact that survival chances may be much better at a specialised hospital. A vociferous CHC and local newspaper has bump started Cancer Specialisation in my Trust. The appointment of a Breast Cancer Surgeon to set up a one-stop clinic was joyously received and stalled criticism. I suspect that there will be more than this. The NHS R&D Directorate and Health Authorities will use public education about relative outcomes to mobilise consumer forces that will accelerate changes in professional practice and provision. All, of course, will favour concentration only of that part of the treatment process whose concentration improves outcome. They will insist on local convenience wherever possible to maintain a treatment programme devised after diagnosis in the specialist centre.

Trusts, especially small ones that will not enter into partnerships with other Trusts, will not prosper. Health Authorities are specifying that joint bids by small Trusts are essential if they are to be granted Cancer Unit status.

9.4.4 Empty achievements

If there are quality improvements to be made by concentration, and perhaps cost savings as well, very clear objectives have to be defined and carefully tracked to ensure that they are delivered. A bigger critical mass of consultants with adequate junior cover will fail to achieve improvements in cost-effectiveness if there is poor leadership and teamwork. It is fine in theory to have greater expertise with sub-specialisation in General Surgery. But if both specialists in upper GI cancers are away at the same time, or there is failure to agree a hospital protocol, what hope is there of improving quality? If larger groupings of specialists do not lead to more effective audit of outcomes, or are not supported by management action to implement the required changes, the point of the exercise is lost. If doctors will not work shift systems so that there is consultant-level specialist advice, twenty-four hours a day, seven days a week, then patients are no better off than they were with dispersed services.

9.4.5 A conundrum

All this drive for sub-specialisation and concentration could have some as yet unexplored disadvantages. The passing of the general physician and general surgeon may deprive patients of a quick diagnosis (always a probability) and a low-tech plan of action (often safe and sufficient). We could end up with super-specialists each able to tell you with authority what you do not have wrong with you, but none able to have a shot at telling you what you do have wrong with you. These specialists would all do more tests, take more time, and use more resources. One might be better off with a general physician or general surgeon, especially in an emergency.

I used to be a psychiatrist and know that patients with their GPs make careful choices of psychiatrist on the basis of reputation, gender, and other personal characteristics. The more consultants in a centre of excellence, the more choice perhaps? Not really, as sectorisation in Psychiatry and Geriatrics, and sub-specialisation in Surgery and Medicine can rapidly diminish choice to one consultant. Experience shows that once a group of generalists start to sub-specialise, even though they promise flexibility to allow choice, administrative barriers soon restrict choice. If Health Authorities are to reconcile promotion of choice with promotion of specialisation, then some radical thinking is needed across primary and secondary care. Between the general practitioner and the specialist with a narrow range of skills, we may need to preserve and treasure some general physicians and general surgeons, and work out where their skills are best deployed.

9.4.6 All in the outcomes

In recent years, Trusts have been swept along by the received wisdom that quality correlates with volume. Managers have tussled with consultants who prefer to retain generalist skills. Neither side has had much evidence to support its arguments. Now we are beginning to learn that the correlation is more specific to conditions and situations. It is great to know that outcomes for leaking aortic aneurysms are hundreds of percent better in a tertiary centre – but only if you are likely to get there alive. I would be prepared to take bets that a particularly gifted surgeon who does these operations relatively infrequently has outcomes equal to a teaching centre. But in the future we shall no doubt have to have such statistics ready for inspection. It was the condition of appointment for an oral surgeon that he would audit and compare his outcomes for complex facio-maxillary operations with surgeons in the tertiary centre. He does and there is no pussy-footedness about 'confidential' audit. The numbers treated by this surgeon may be less important than ensuring that before he starts this work the hospital is adequately equipped. Outcomes may well depend on the adequacy of support services like intensive care and radiological imaging.

Trusts do have to manage, much more carefully than in the past, the introduction of new procedures. It was something of a shock to some of our surgeons to realise that the Trust Board would not accept medical indemnity for a surgeon starting to carry out a new operation without following the Trust's procedures for ensuring cost-effectiveness, appropriate training, required facilities and of course purchaser agreement. The management–professional relationships may be a critical factor in determining whether high and low-volume centres produce better or worse outcomes for particular conditions. Surgeons in a Trust like mine might well obtain good outcomes with a surgeon treating low volumes of patients if the management back-up is of a high order. What is called intensive care in one Trust may have very different standards from that in another. Most of the cost savings made by concentrating services appear to be obtained through avoiding the multiplication of back-up services. There has been plenty of that in my area, with all Trusts having CT scanners working at well below 50 per cent capacity.

9.4.7 The final determinant is money

With Trusts increasingly desperate to find ways of achieving financial viability it is no wonder that they behave like whores. We do whatever the punter likes. Our problem is making sense of the confusing, contradictory requirements of multiple fundholding practices. Quite often what they say they want is at variance with what they do want. Noble talk about seeking quality must be tested against the facts of seeking the shortest waiting time however bad the reputation of another hospital, or going for a lower price after inviting a Trust to provide expensive local clinics.

After a period of fairly vigorous growth in all specialties, Trusts are now facing cuts in elective care to fund the continued rise in emergencies. Reducing spare capacity and fixed costs will be more difficult if spread across many Trusts. This could be another drive for more concentration to reduce costs.

Where there is to be concentration the public will need to understand why. Much better public relations will be required to involve communities, and patients within communities, in deciding what they really want in terms of concentration and localisation of services. It will require sophisticated public relations led by Health Authorities to orchestrate GPs and consultants in handling these messages so that the public can understand the issues rather than be confused and frightened by the arguments.

GPs now tell us that many patients will opt to travel large distances for better treatment where they can rely on easy car-parking. Trusts like mine must carefully consider large capital investment in multi-storey car-parking. There could be a double bonus, in attracting patients and generating income because people are getting used to paying to park at hospitals. Car-parks are steady earners.

9.4.8 In conclusion

I suggest that purchasers, in choosing which Trust will grow and which Trust will shrink, should take much more account of the management–professional relationship and how it impacts on the teamwork and co-ordination of facilities required for safe and effective treatment of patients. This may be a more important factor in cost-effectiveness than high volume and pushing sub-specialisation to its limits. Before the generalist physicians and surgeons disappear or lose status, more careful consideration needs to be given to their roles. We may be losing skills of great importance to the welfare of patients and the conservation of resources.

The real challenge for Trusts is to develop specialists into team players, against traditions which have been highly individualist. Consultant appointments committees need to be as interested in management and team-leadership qualities, as in technical abilities. If this is done well professionals will find their work less stressful and more satisfying as part of a team. And Trusts themselves must be team players, forming alliances with other Trusts to provide the best specialist and local services for patients. Perhaps, we might see Trusts competing to be nice to each other in striving to retain contracts with Health Authorities!

REFERENCES: THE LEGAL FRAMEWORK

Allen P 1995 Contracts in the National Health Service Internal Market. Modern Law Review 58 (3) 321–342.

Appleby J 1994 Developing Contracting. National Association of Health Authorities and Trusts, Birmingham.

Attiyah P 1979 The Rise and Fall of Freedom of Contract. Clarendon Press, Oxford.

Dawson D 1994 Costs and Prices in the Internal Market: Markets vs the NHS. Management Executive Guidelines. Discussion Paper 115. Centre for Health Economics, University of York, York.

Dawson D 1995 Regulating Competition in the NHS: The Department of Health Guide on Mergers and Anti-Competitive Behaviour Discussion Paper 131. Centre for Health Economics, University of York: York.

Guesnerie R 1989 Hidden Actions, Moral Hazard and Contract Theory. In Eatwell J, Milgate M and P Newman (eds) Allocation, Information and Markets. Macmillan: London.

Hughes D and Dingwall R 1990 Sir Henry Maine, Joseph Stalin and the Reorganisation of the NHS. Journal of Social Welfare Law: 5.

Hughes D, McHale J and Griffiths L 1994 NHS Arbitration – a Redundant Remedy. Paper given at ESRC Contracts and Competition Programme Workshop, Robinson College, Cambridge University.

Jacob J 1991 Lawyers go to Hospital. Public Law: 255–281.

National Health Service Contracts (Dispute Resolution) Regulations Statutory Instrument 1996 No 623.

National Health Service Executive 1994 The Operation of the NHS Internal Market: Local Freedoms, National Responsibilities. HSG(94)55 National Health Service Executive, Leeds.

National Health Service Management Executive 1990 NHS Trusts: A Working Guide. National Health Service Management Executive, Leeds.

National Health Service Management Executive 1991 NHS Contracts: Guidance on Resolving Disputes. EL (91) 11.

National Health Service Executive 1997 Changing the Internal Market. EL (97) 33.

REFERENCES: ACCOUNTABILITY AND HEALTHCARE MARKETS

Committee of Public Accounts 1993 Wessex Regional Health Authority Regional Information Systems Plan. London, HMSO.

Committee of Public Accounts 1994 The Proper Conduct of Public Business. London, HMSO.

Dawson D 1995 Regulating Competition in the NHS: The Department of Health Guide on Mergers and Anti-Competitive Behaviour. University of York, Centre for Health Economics Discussion Paper 131.

Day P, Klein R 1987 Accountabilities: Five Public Services. London, Tavistock.

Department of Health 1994 Operation of the NHS Internal Market: Local Freedoms, National Responsibilities. London, Department of Health.

Dunleavy P, Hood C 1994 From Old Public Administration to New Public Management. Public Money and Management 14(3): 9–17.

Ferlie E, Ashburner L, Fitzgerald L, Pettigrew A 1996 The New Public Management in Action. Oxford, Oxford University Press.

Foot M 1973 Aneurin Bevan. Volume II, 1945–60. London, Davis-Poynter.

Lowndes V 1996 The New Institutionalism: A Critical Appraisal. Public Administration 74;181–97.

Mays N, Dixon J 1996 Purchaser Plurality in UK Health Care. London, King's Fund.

National Audit Office 1996a Health of the Nation: A Progress Report. London, HMSO.

National Audit Office 1996b NHS Supplies. London, HMSO.

National Audit Office 1996c Health and Safety in Hospitals. London, HMSO.

National Audit Office 1996d The Regulation of Gas Tariffs: The Gas Cost Index. London, HMSO.

NHS Executive 1994 Code of Conduct and Accountability. Leeds, NHS Executive.

Ogus A 1994 Regulation: Legal Form and Economic Theory. Oxford, Oxford University Press.

Osborne D, Gaebler T 1992 Reinventing Government. Reading, Massachusetts, Addison-Wesley.

Pollitt C 1993 Managerialism and the Public Services. Second Edition. Oxford, Blackwell.

10

Epilogue: service development under uncertainty

In 1996 the NHS Executive commissioned the University of York (NHS Centre for Reviews and Dissemination, Centre for Health Economics and the York Health Economics Consortium) to undertake several reviews which form the basis of Chapters 2–5 of this book. The NHS Executive was prompted to commission the work by the number of local proposals for organisational change and for capital development that seemed to be founded upon questionable assumptions regarding the most efficient and effective structure of healthcare delivery, and by the hope that Health Authorities and others involved in local configuration proposals would welcome a survey of the available evidence.

Notwithstanding the York reviews, the extent of ignorance regarding most of the key factors that should determine optimal service and organisational configuration remains daunting. This Chapter is mainly devoted to sketching the extent of this uncertainty, but draws some tentative conclusions – particularly suggesting that health-service commissioners can ease their burden by differentiating between decisions that are properly theirs from those that are best taken by providers.

10.1 FIVE QUESTIONABLE ASSUMPTIONS

Five questionable assumptions in the planning of service re-configurations have proved particularly prevalent.

First, the assumption that **savings can come through organisational merger, irrespective of whether a reduction in capital capacity will follow.** The merging of two organisations, it is often averred, will lead to the automatic saving of the Board costs of one of them. The obvious but often overlooked danger is that putting two organisations together will in fact lead to the creation of a management superstructure on top of existing management.

Evidence is provided in Chapter 3 that hospital scale efficiencies are exhausted in the 300–500 bed range, and that inefficiencies start to creep in for sites above this range. If a large single hospital is less efficient than a small single hospital, it is likely (though not certain) that a large multi-site hospital will be less efficient than several single site hospitals. In the NHS this hypothesis is partly substantiated by reports from multi-site hospital Trusts of substantial costs associated with managing across sites.

The direct evidence of the effectiveness of mergers in the NHS, or in other health systems, is weak. However, the evidence base for mergers in other industries is much richer and supports scepticism regarding the value that is added by mergers. The problem in other sectors is thought to lie with the corporate governance system: dispersed shareholders are unable to prevent executives from launching take-overs that add to their own power and remuneration without increasing shareholder value. In the NHS the position of the shareholder with the veto on such proposals is played by the NHS Executive. The moral of the comparison is that the Executive should be wary of local enthusiasm for merger proposals.

This is not to deny that there are efficient multi-hospital systems, just as there are efficient large hospitals: exceptional individuals and circumstances can prevail against the generality. And indeed there is no strong evidence that mergers cannot yield efficiency or quality gains. The point is that there is no rule that indicates that organisational or site merger will generate savings. Each case must be evaluated on its merits.

Some merger proposals presented as likely to yield cost economies may actually be motivated by two other concerns. Capacity reductions may be more easily secured – more easily from a political or managerial perspective – through merger. Alternatively, it could be that

one management team is much stronger than another.

The second assumption is that **short-term savings arising from merger will be sustained irrespective of lost contestability.** Commissioners are often aware that a merger proposal they are supporting will reduce their leverage, but short-term financial pressures may lead them to discount the medium-term costs of lost leverage. Furthermore, the loss of efficiency and responsiveness consequent upon reduced contestability are very hard to quantify, and what is not quantified tends to be ignored.

Third is the assumption that **clinical quality and outcomes are enhanced by concentration.** The York review addressed this directly and revealed that there is robust evidence of volume–quality links in only a minority of cases, and in some of those there is evidence that the volume–quality links run out at modest levels (Chapter 2). Even where there is evidence of volume–quality links the direction of causation is not established. It may be that the best doctors are attracting the largest case-loads, or perhaps that the best doctors get jobs at the largest hospitals. Such explanations of a volume–quality link would indicate that increased quality might not be secured merely by combining smaller, poorer quality Trusts.

But even where there are volume-quality links *and* the causation is of a practice-makes-perfect variety (which might support merger proposals), there may be clinical and other patient costs of concentration offsetting the benefits. Important factors are:

- the distance-decay relationship, which was investigated in the York study (see Chapter 4): i.e. worse clinical outcomes due to reduced access;
- increased patient travel time and cost;
- inappropriate allocation to sub-specialists. Sub-specialisation may well yield increased quality and outcomes for those patients who are appropriately targeted to the sub-specialists. However, in the field of medical emergency particularly, there is increasing concern amongst the clinicians and Royal Colleges that the loss of generalist capacity to diagnose and treat illnesses that are diffi-

cult to allocate to a sub-specialty, or where there are multiple co-morbidities, may lead to adverse outcomes. If it turns out that more generalists are required to undertake initial diagnosis of medical emergencies (for example), then smaller hospitals may turn out to be clinically viable – so long as there are adequate professional and transport links to referral centres.

Fourth, **clinical specialisation and linkages are often assumed to require an organisational merger.** Both commissioners and providers have tended to assume that the current framework of NHS acute provision, organised around single or multiple hospital Trusts, is immutable. Hence, where clinical linkage has been required for quality or training purposes, Trust merger has been proposed. Yet clinical linkages across Trusts could be developed, in protocols or in contracts, neither compromising the independence of the operational management of Trusts, nor precipitating merger of all clinical functions. Technological developments such as telemedicine could facilitate such solutions.

More generally, the determination of optimal organisational form requires separate analysis from that designed to establish the optimal size of hospital or of clinical teams. Optimal organisational scale will vary with demography, geography, communications links, complexity and heterogeneity of services.

One key question here is: should the organisation delivering the service also own the assets from where the services are delivered? If it should, the sunk costs involved will deter entry. Many industries have seen the separation of management of infrastructure from that of service providers precisely in order to allow new entry and contestability (e.g. airports, the National Grid, BT's network, Railtrack). Such models could in theory be implemented locally in the NHS. These models all involve the creation of contractual links between the infrastructure owners/managers and the service providers.

The fifth assumption is that **Royal College training specifications are indefeasible.** Often Royal Colleges will set a target for throughput which is indicative rather than prescriptive. Discussions with Royal Colleges, as part of the York study, have revealed that they are not setting out to dictate the pattern of hospital configuration. On the contrary they are aiming to develop training systems that are robust. Given the limited available evidence regarding the effectiveness of particular training patterns, it is reasonable that training should in general be fitted around systems designed to meet service quality and efficiency objectives.

10.2 LOCATING DECISIONS WITH THOSE WITH ADEQUATE INFORMATION AND APPROPRIATE INCENTIVES

These assumptions are questionable because of a lack of general evidence upon which to make generalisations regarding the organisation of healthcare. This lack of general information, together with an asymmetry in the distribution of local information (the providers have much of the relevant information) has profound implications for the optimal location of decision-making between commissioners and providers.

The factors that should be taken into account when assessing local re-configuration proposals include the following:

- **Efficient hospital scale**, i.e. how large (number of beds, or interventions, or patients treated) should a hospital be? (The York study provided evidence on acute hospitals; but there is uncertainty about the efficient scale for community hospitals; and even the acute studies may be superseded by shifting boundaries between the community and acute, and between primary and community, and by technical change.)
- **Optimal organisational scale**, i.e. how large an organisation should run health services (from a multi-hospital system at one extreme, to independent clinical departments at the other)? If a large system is optimal, what incentives will remain to improve efficiency and quality? Should clinical services and facilities be managed together or separately?
- **Volume-outcome links**, i.e. will there be clinical benefits to the patients treated if they are treated in the same unit? How do benefits from greater sub-specialist proficiency

balance against loss of access, higher patient transport costs and loss of generalist diagnostic skills?

- **Inter-speciality linkages**, i.e. which specialties need to be co-located, and for which do organisational or transport links need to be developed?
- **Transition costs**, i.e. what are the capital, staff and morale costs of setting new systems in place? What are the equivalent costs of maintaining the status quo?
- **Flexibility**, i.e. how robust is the proposal against epidemiological and technological change?

In the absence of rules of thumb, let alone robust generalisations, regarding most of these factors, decision-makers are forced to rely upon painstaking assessments of the local environment and the particular consequences of proposals for the health of local populations.

The Health Authority, or other Health Commissioners, has been expected to assess proposals, and to underwrite or ratify plans. Yet, faced with a re-configuration or capital investment proposal, commissioners are in a very weak position to gather the requisite local information to determine whether the proposal offers value for money relative to the status quo, let alone relative to the (unknown) best alternative. It is not surprising under such pressures that commissioners are driven to make bold, but questionable, assumptions or to go along with the plans proposed by providers.

The corollary is that health service commissioners should eschew the rôle of ratifier and implicit guarantor of provider re-organisations and capital plans, because:

- most of the critical information about costs of re-configuration proposals lies within the provider sector: purchasers have found themselves reliant upon advice from local stakeholders, critically including the providers themselves, in determining which capital and organisational projects to sponsor;
- the advice given by providers in these circumstances cannot be disinterested. Providers have a vested interest in under-stating the gains that could be made *without* new investment or concentration, and of

over-stating the gains that can be made *with* such investment;
- if commissioners take responsibility for ratifying or commissioning capital or organisational change, they thereby remove responsibility from the providers for achieving change within the budget set.

The commissioner's rôle might rather be to specify with the maximum of clarity and financial commitment, the healthcare requirements of it's population for the coming years. Health Authority and primary-care commissioners could determine the likely call on the secondary sector, and then offer medium-term financial commitments for the treatment of patients in different need categories to specified (though negotiable) quality standards.

It would be for the providers, thus challenged by the commissioners' needs and service specifications, to gather information on the costs of different configurations of provision, and to formulate proposals. They could then respond to commissioners by detailing the costs, outcomes and quality that their preferred method and location of delivery can offer. Purchasers would sign up to, and hold providers to account for, the quality and price of services delivered, not the configuration of supply.

Providers might judge that certain investments or reorganisations would be necessary to deliver the most effective and efficient solution. Where capital is required for such reorganisation, the contracts on offer from commissioners would form the security against which public or private funders would invest. (Some investments will be attractive only on the basis of returns beyond the term of any funding agreements that commissioners are willing to sign. In such cases, scrutiny by either the private sector funders, or Government, would have to be particularly intense.)

Whether or not capital is required, the NHS needs to develop the flexibility to allow reorganisation to match commissioner specifications, rather than fitting patient care around existing institutional structures.

Negotiations might cover the risk allocation between purchaser and provider for volume variation, minimum quality standards, access and other issues. Assigning financial risk for volume variation to commissioners, for example, whilst giving providers responsibility for achieving the cost and quality benchmarks, would reward commissioners (both Health Authority and primary-care commissioners) for minimising the call on the secondary sector, and reward providers for achieving quality targets at lower than forecast cost.

There is an additional reason for wishing providers rather than purchasers to make the decisions and commitments on reorganisation, concentration and capital: the nexus between the 'three markets' – for healthcare, for training and for research. There is no reason to suppose that the optimal configuration for healthcare delivery will coincide with that for training or for research.

The independent funding streams that now support these activities were put in place with just such possibilities in mind. Providers contemplating capital or organisational development can take account of all three funding streams in assessing the merits of different options. Funders of development capital should equally balance the costs and benefits of different proposals for delivering services in each of the three markets.

The healthcare commissioner, by contrast, trying to make the same judgement, would find him or herself not only trying to second-guess the achievable costs and quality in healthcare, research and training services, where expertise resides with the provider, but would also have to second-guess the priorities and budgets of the commissioners of training and research. Either that or the health commissioner would have to collaborate with the training and research commissioners in a configuration review that would become unwieldy in the extreme.

A final reason for locating responsibility for organisational proposals with providers is the interplay between the organisation of healthcare and the medical labour market. A common driver towards merger is the difficulty of attracting new staff to existing posts, together with the need to adapt to reduced junior doctor hours and new training arrangements. Providers, particularly if clinicians are closely

involved in the development of proposals, are in a much stronger position than commissioners to design flexible mechanisms for addressing these problems in ways that are consistent with the maintenance of quality, access and efficiency.

The one strategic issue related to the organisation of healthcare delivery that is not directly related to quality, access and price, yet upon which the commissioner might wish to take a view, is the question of contestable form. Even if the proposed reorganisation promises high-quality, low-cost services, is there a danger that when it comes to contract renewal the commissioner will be left without leverage? To avoid that outcome, commissioners may wish to negotiate discrete agreements for different services, and give preference to smaller organisations working constructively with each other over larger monolithic enterprises.

How does this model for provider-led development of capital or reorganisation fit with the shift towards strategic collaboration, which the Government is now seeking to engender between purchasers and providers within the NHS?

Identifying the purchaser's role as that of standing back from provider configuration issues and challenging providers to come up with different proposals to deliver high-quality, low-cost care, actually fits very well with a more strategic collaboration between purchasers and providers.

One key change that the Government has promised is the extension of the term of funding agreements that commissioners will be offering. Longer-term funding agreements offer providers security upon which to make cost and quality commitments, and security upon which to undertake capital and human investment (and some security upon which to secure the requisite transitional funding).

The annuality of the contracting cycle – itself a reflection of risk aversion in the system – has left providers unwilling or unable to commit themselves to reorganisation and investment, changes which could have yielded significant cost savings in the medium term. With providers unable to make such commitments, it has paradoxically fallen to purchasers to organise service reviews, and then to propose and endorse capital and organisational proposals which commit large elements of their budgets for many years, often on the basis of very questionable assumptions and biased local information. More robust commitments by com-

missioners regarding health needs and resulting service specifications, based on the best available evidence, would enable and encourage providers to take responsibility for the risks that they can best manage: those related to organisational and capital configuration.

Index

When added to a page number f denotes a term in a figure and t denotes a term in a table.